# Guidance for Establishing Crisis Standards of Care for Use in Disaster Situations

## A Letter Report

Committee on Guidance for Establishing Standards of Care for Use in Disaster Situations

Board on Health Sciences Policy

Bruce M. Altevogt, Clare Stroud, Sarah L. Hanson, Dan Hanfling, and Lawrence O. Gostin, *Editors*

INSTITUTE OF MEDICINE
OF THE NATIONAL ACADEMIES

THE NATIONAL ACADEMIES PRESS
Washington, D.C.
**www.nap.edu**

**THE NATIONAL ACADEMIES PRESS • 500 Fifth Street, N.W. • Washington, DC 20001**

NOTICE: The project that is the subject of this report was approved by the Governing Board of the National Research Council, whose members are drawn from the councils of the National Academy of Sciences, the National Academy of Engineering, and the Institute of Medicine. The members of the committee responsible for the report were chosen for their special competences and with regard for appropriate balance.

This study was requested by the Office of the Assistant Secretary for Preparedness and Response, Department of Health and Human Services, and supported by Contract No. HHSP23320042509XI between the National Academy of Sciences and the Department of Health and Human Services. Any opinions, findings, conclusions, or recommendations expressed in this publication are those of the author(s) and do not necessarily reflect the view of the organizations or agencies that provided support for this project.

International Standard Book Number-13: 978-0-309-14430-8
International Standard Book Number-11: 0-309-14430-2

Additional copies of this report are available from the National Academies Press, 500 Fifth Street, N.W., Lockbox 285, Washington, DC 20055; (800) 624-6242 or (202) 334-3313 (in the Washington metropolitan area); Internet, http://www.nap.edu.

For more information about the Institute of Medicine, visit the IOM home page at: **www.iom.edu.**

Printed in the United States of America

Suggested citation: IOM (Institute of Medicine). 2009. *Guidance for establishing crisis standards of care for use in disaster situations: A letter report.* Washington, DC: The National Academies Press.

# THE NATIONAL ACADEMIES
*Advisers to the Nation on Science, Engineering, and Medicine*

The **National Academy of Sciences** is a private, nonprofit, self-perpetuating society of distinguished scholars engaged in scientific and engineering research, dedicated to the furtherance of science and technology and to their use for the general welfare. Upon the authority of the charter granted to it by the Congress in 1863, the Academy has a mandate that requires it to advise the federal government on scientific and technical matters. Dr. Ralph J. Cicerone is president of the National Academy of Sciences.

The **National Academy of Engineering** was established in 1964, under the charter of the National Academy of Sciences, as a parallel organization of outstanding engineers. It is autonomous in its administration and in the selection of its members, sharing with the National Academy of Sciences the responsibility for advising the federal government. The National Academy of Engineering also sponsors engineering programs aimed at meeting national needs, encourages education and research, and recognizes the superior achievements of engineers. Dr. Charles M. Vest is president of the National Academy of Engineering.

The **Institute of Medicine** was established in 1970 by the National Academy of Sciences to secure the services of eminent members of appropriate professions in the examination of policy matters pertaining to the health of the public. The Institute acts under the responsibility given to the National Academy of Sciences by its congressional charter to be an adviser to the federal government and, upon its own initiative, to identify issues of medical care, research, and education. Dr. Harvey V. Fineberg is president of the Institute of Medicine.

The **National Research Council** was organized by the National Academy of Sciences in 1916 to associate the broad community of science and technology with the Academy's purposes of furthering knowledge and advising the federal government. Functioning in accordance with general policies determined by the Academy, the Council has become the principal operating agency of both the National Academy of Sciences and the National Academy of Engineering in providing services to the government, the public, and the scientific and engineering communities. The Council is administered jointly by both Academies and the Institute of Medicine. Dr. Ralph J. Cicerone and Dr. Charles M. Vest are chair and vice chair, respectively, of the National Research Council.

**www.national-academies.org**

*"Knowing is not enough; we must apply.*
*Willing is not enough; we must do."*
—Goethe

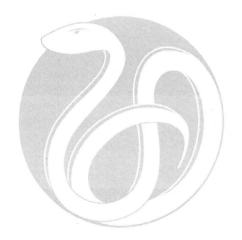

# INSTITUTE OF MEDICINE
*OF THE NATIONAL ACADEMIES*

**Advising the Nation. Improving Health.**

**COMMITTEE ON GUIDANCE FOR ESTABLISHING
STANDARDS OF CARE FOR USE IN DISASTER SITUATIONS**

**LAWRENCE O. GOSTIN** (*Chair*), Georgetown University Law Center
**DAN HANFLING** (*Vice Chair*), Inova Health System
**DAMON T. ARNOLD,** Department of Public Health, Illinois
**STEPHEN V. CANTRILL,** Denver Health Medical Center
**BROOKE COURTNEY,** Center for Biosecurity of the University of
  Pittsburgh Medical Center
**ASHA DEVEREAUX,** Sharp Coronado Hospital, CA
**EDWARD J. GABRIEL,** The Walt Disney Company
**JOHN L. HICK,** Hennepin County Medical Center
**JAMES G. HODGE, JR.,** Sandra Day O'Connor College of Law at
  Arizona State University
**DONNA E. LEVIN,** Massachusetts Department of Public Health
**MARIANNE MATZO,** University of Oklahoma College of Nursing
**CHERYL A. PETERSON,** American Nurses Association
**TIA POWELL,** Montefiore-Einstein Center for Bioethics, Bronx
**MERRITT SCHREIBER,** UCLA Center for Public Health and
  Disasters
**UMAIR A. SHAH,** Harris County Public Health and Environmental
  Service, Houston, TX

*Study Staff*

**BRUCE M. ALTEVOGT,** Study Director
**CATHARYN T. LIVERMAN,** Scholar
**ANDREW M. POPE,** Director, Board on Health Sciences Policy
**SARAH L. HANSON,** Associate Program Officer
**CLARE STROUD,** Associate Program Officer
**JON SANDERS,** Program Associate

# Reviewers

This report has been reviewed in draft form by individuals chosen for their diverse perspectives and technical expertise, in accordance with procedures approved by the National Research Council's Report Review Committee. The purpose of this independent review is to provide candid and critical comments that will assist the institution in making its published report as sound as possible and to ensure that the report meets institutional standards for objectivity, evidence, and responsiveness to the study charge. The review comments and draft manuscript remain confidential to protect the integrity of the deliberative process. We wish to thank the following individuals for their review of this report:

**Frederick M. Burkle Jr.,** University of Hawaii
**Kristine M. Gebbie,** Hunter College City University, New York
**Steven Gravely,** Troutman Sanders, LLP
**Sharona Hoffman,** Case Western Reserve University
**Lisa Kaplowitz,** Virginia Department of Health
**Gabor D. Kelen,** Johns Hopkins University School of Medicine
**Nancie McAnaugh,** Missouri Department of Health and
    Services
**Leslee Stein-Spencer,** National Association of State EMS Officials
**Matthew K. Wynia,** American Medical Association

Although the reviewers listed above have provided many constructive comments and suggestions, they were not asked to endorse the conclusions or recommendations, nor did they see the final draft of the report before its release. The review of this report was overseen by **Bernard Lo,** University of California, San Francisco and

**Georges Benjamin,** American Public Health Association. Appointed by the National Research Council and Institute of Medicine, they were responsible for making certain that an independent examination of this report was carried out in accordance with institutional procedures and that all review comments were carefully considered. Responsibility for the final content of this report rests entirely with the authoring committee and the institution.

# Contents

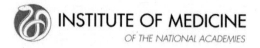

**INSTITUTE OF MEDICINE**
OF THE NATIONAL ACADEMIES

September 24, 2009

Nicole Lurie, M.D., M.S.P.H.
Assistant Secretary for Preparedness
  and Response
Office of the Assistant Secretary for
  Preparedness and Response
Department of Health and Human Services
200 Independence Ave., S.W.
Washington, DC 20201

Dear Dr. Lurie:

On behalf of the Institute of Medicine (IOM) Committee on Guidance for Establishing Standards of Care for Use in Disaster Situations, we are pleased to report our conclusions and recommendations. At the request of the Office of the Assistant Secretary for Preparedness and Response, Department of Health and Human Services, the IOM convened this committee to develop guidance that state and local public health officials and health-sector agencies and institutions can use to establish and implement standards of care that should apply in disaster situations—both naturally occurring and manmade—under scarce resource conditions. Specifically, the committee was asked to identify and describe the key elements that should be included in standards of care protocols, to identify potential triggers, and to develop a template matrix that can be used by state and local public health officials as a framework for developing specific guidance for healthcare provider communities to develop crisis standards of care. The committee was asked to consider the roles and responsibilities of various stakeholders in the implementation of the guidance, and to consider mechanisms for integrating the views of the general public and healthcare providers in the development and implementation of the guidance. The committee was also specifically charged with incorporating ethical principles into the guidance.

To accomplish its charge within the accelerated time frame, the committee held a 4-day meeting that included a 1-day workshop. Panel discussions at the workshop focused on federal and state efforts associated with establishing standards of care; guidance on standards of care in medical triage events; changing roles and responsibilities of healthcare workers under contingency and crisis standards of care; guidance on legal, ethical, and practical issues in setting standards of care in declared emergencies; and identifying triggers. The committee does seek to make clear that the extraordinary time constraints significantly limited the opportunity to consider more evidence and enlist other stakeholders in the deliberations process. This is particularly true given the complexity and importance of the issues being considered. This letter serves as a summary of the committee's conclusions and recommendations. Greater detail can be found in the relevant report text that follows this letter.

Through a careful review of available protocols, the committee recognizes that although some federal, state, municipality, territorial, and health-sector agencies and institutions have made considerable progress in developing protocols, many states have only just begun to address this urgent need. Furthermore, there is a need to develop all protocols around the same key elements and components to ensure coordination, consistency, and fair allocation of scarce resources during a disaster.

In the development of its national guidance on standards of care, the committee was asked to consider if there should be a single national guidance or scenario-specific guidance. Based on a review of the currently available state standards of care protocols, published literature, and testimony provided at its workshop, the committee concluded that there is an urgent and clear need for a single national guidance for states for crisis standards of care that can be generalized to all crisis events and is not specific to a certain event. However, the committee recognizes that within the single general framework, individual disaster scenarios may require specific considerations, such as differences between no-notice events versus slow-onset events, but that the key elements and components remain the same.

The committee was tasked to develop national framework guidance on the key elements that should be included in standards of care protocols for disaster situations. Ethical norms in medical care do not change during disasters – health care professionals are always obligated to provide the best care they reasonably can under given circumstances. For purposes of developing recommendations for situations when healthcare resources are overwhelmed, the committee defines the level of health and medical care capable of being delivered during a catastrophic event as *crisis standards of care*.

"Crisis standards of care" is defined as a substantial change in usual healthcare operations and the level of care it is possible to deliver, which is made necessary by a pervasive (e.g., pandemic influenza) or catastrophic (e.g., earthquake, hurricane) disaster. This change in the level of care delivered is justified by specific circumstances and is formally declared by a state government, in recognition that crisis operations will be in effect for a sustained period. The formal declaration that crisis standards of care are in operation enables specific legal/regulatory powers and protections for healthcare providers in the necessary tasks of allocating and using scarce medical resources and implementing alternate care facility operations.

To ensure that the utmost care possible is provided to patients in a catastrophic event, the nation needs a robust system to guide the public, healthcare professionals and institutions, and governmental entities at all levels. To achieve such a system of just care, the committee sets forth the following vision for crisis standards of care:

- *Fairness*—standards that are, to the highest degree possible, recognized as fair by all those affected by them – including the members of affected communities, practitioners, and provider organizations, evidence based and responsive to specific needs of individuals and the population focused on a duty of compassion and care, a duty to steward resources, and a goal of maintaining the trust of patients and the community
- *Equitable processes*—processes and procedures for ensuring that decisions and implementation of standards are made equitably
    - *Transparency*—in design and decision making
    - *Consistency*—in application across populations and among individuals regardless of their human condition (e.g., race, age, disability, ethnicity, ability to pay, socioeconomic status, preexisting health conditions, social worth, perceived obstacles to treatment, past use of resources)
    - *Proportionality*—public and individual requirements must be commensurate with the scale of the emergency and degree of scarce resources

      o  *Accountability*—of individuals deciding and implementing standards, and of governments for ensuring appropriate protections and just allocation of available resources
- *Community and provider engagement, education, and communication*—active collaboration with the public and stakeholders for their input is essential through formalized processes
- *The rule of law*
  - o  *Authority*—to empower necessary and appropriate actions and interventions in response to emergencies
  - o  *Environment*—to facilitate implementation through laws that support standards and create appropriate incentives

Throughout the report the committee emphasizes the need for states to develop and implement consistent crisis standards of care protocols both within the state and through work with neighboring states, in collaboration with their partners in the public and private sectors. This report contains guidance to assist state public health authorities in developing these crisis standards of care. This guidance includes criteria for determining when crisis standards of care should be implemented, key elements that should be included in the crisis standards of care protocols, and criteria for determining when these standards of care should be implemented.

With the intent of assisting the many states that are still in the early stages of developing crisis standards of care, the committee lays out a broad process for developing crisis standards of care protocols that encompasses the full spectrum of the health system, including emergency medical services and dispatch, public health, hospital-based care, home care, primary care, palliative care, mental health, and public health. Furthermore, although the compressed time frame limited the scope of the work presented here and the opportunity for a robust community-engagement process, the committee strongly recommends extensive engagement with community and provider stakeholders. Such public engagement is necessary not only to ensure the legitimacy of the process and standards, but more importantly to achieve the best possible result.

> **Recommendation: <u>Develop Consistent State Crisis Standards of Care Protocols with Five Key Elements</u>**
> **State departments of health, and other relevant state agencies, in partnership with localities should develop crisis standards of care protocols that include**

the key elements—and associated components—
detailed in this report:

- A strong ethical grounding;
- Integrated and ongoing community and provider engagement, education, and communication;
- Assurances regarding legal authority and environment;
- Clear indicators, triggers, and lines of responsibility; and
- Evidence-based clinical processes and operations.

**Recommendation: <u>Seek Community and Provider
Engagement</u>**
State, local, and tribal governments should partner
with and work to ensure strong public engagement of
community and provider stakeholders, with particular attention given to the needs of vulnerable populations and those with medical special needs, in:

- Developing and refining crisis standards of
  care protocols and implementation guidance;
- Creating and disseminating educational tools
  and messages to both the public and health
  professionals;
- Developing and implementing crisis communication strategies;
- Developing and implementing community resilience strategies; and
- Learning from and improving crisis standards of care response situations.

An ethical framework serves as the bedrock for public policy and
cannot be added as an afterthought. Hence, ethical principles underlie the
committee's vision for crisis planning, outlined above. In addition, ethically and clinically sound planning will aim to secure fair and equitable
resources and protections for vulnerable groups. The committee concluded that core ethical precepts in medicine permit some actions during

crisis situations that would not be acceptable under ordinary circumstances, such as implementing resource allocation protocols that could preclude the use of certain resources on some patients when others would derive greater benefit from them. But even here, it is the situation that changes during disasters, not ethical standards *per se*. The context of a disaster may make certain resources unavailable for some or even all patients, but it does not provide license to act without regard to professional or legal standards. Healthcare professionals are obligated always to provide the best care they reasonably can to each patient in their care, including during crises. When resource scarcity reaches catastrophic levels, clinicians are ethically justified – and indeed are ethically obligated – to use the available resources to sustain life and well-being to the greatest extent possible. As a result, the committee concluded that ethics permits clinicians to allocate scarce resources so as to provide necessary and available treatments preferentially to those patients most likely to benefit when operating under crisis standards of care. However, operating under crisis standards of care does not permit clinicians to ignore professional norms nor to act without ethical standards or accountability.

> **Recommendation: <u>Adhere to Ethical Norms During Crisis Standards of Care</u>**
> **When crisis standards of care prevail, as when ordinary standards are in effect, healthcare practitioners must adhere to ethical norms. Conditions of overwhelming scarcity limit autonomous choices for both patients and practitioners regarding the allocation of scarce healthcare resources, but do not permit actions that violate ethical norms.**

The committee also addressed issues related to the implementation of standards of care, including legal considerations. Questions of legal empowerment of various actions to protect individual and communal health are pervasive and complicated by interjurisdictional inconsistencies. The law should clarify prevailing standards of care and create incentives for actors to respond to protect the public's health and respect individual rights.

**Recommendation: <u>Provide Necessary Legal Protec-
tions for Healthcare Practitioners and Institutions
Implementing Crisis Standards of Care</u>**
**In disaster situations, tribal or state governments
should authorize appropriate agencies to institute
crisis standards of care in affected areas, adjust
scopes of practice for licensed or certified healthcare
practitioners, and alter licensure and credentialing
practices as needed in declared emergencies to create
incentives to provide care needed for the health of
individuals and the public.**

Finally, and continuing the theme of consistency, the committee
highlighted operational issues to ensure the consistent implementation of
the crisis standards of care in a disaster situation within and among
states.

**Recommendation: <u>Ensure Consistency in Crisis
Standards of Care Implementation</u>**
**State departments of health, and other relevant state
agencies, in partnership with localities should ensure
consistent implementation of crisis standards of care
in response to a disaster event. These efforts should
include:**

- **Using "clinical care committees," "triage
  teams," and a state-level "disaster medical
  advisory committee" that will evaluate evidence-based, peer-reviewed critical care and
  other decision tools and recommend and implement decision-making algorithms to be
  used when specific life-sustaining resources
  become scarce;**
- **Providing palliative care services for all patients, including the provision of comfort,
  compassion, and maintenance of dignity;**
- **Mobilizing mental health resources to help
  communities—and providers themselves—to
  manage the effects of crisis standards of care**

**by following a concept of operations developed for disasters;**

- **Developing specific response measures for vulnerable populations and those with medical special needs, including pediatrics, geriatrics, and persons with disabilities; and**

- **Implementing robust situational awareness capabilities to allow for real-time information sharing across affected communities and with the "disaster medical advisory committee."**

**Recommendation: <u>Ensure Intrastate and Interstate Consistency Among Neighboring Jurisdictions</u>**
**States, in partnership with the federal government, tribes, and localities, should initiate communications and develop processes to ensure intrastate and interstate consistency in the implementation of crisis standards of care. Specific efforts are needed to ensure that the Department of Defense, Veterans Health Administration, and Indian Health Services medical facilities are integrated into planning and response efforts.**

The guidance outlined here is intended to assist federal, tribal, state, and local officials in the development of more uniform crisis standards of care policies and protocols that are applicable in any disaster impacting the public's health. Applying the guidance and principles laid out in the report, the committee developed two brief case studies that may serve to illustrate the implementation crisis standards of care. Recognizing the current attention and concern surrounding the 2009 H1N1 pandemic, one scenario focuses on a gradual-onset influenza pandemic modeled around potential issues that may arise this fall during the current pandemic. The second scenario focuses on an earthquake as a model for discussion of the issues that would arise due to a no-notice sudden onset event.

The committee's intent is to provide a framework that allows consistency in establishing the key components required of any effort focused on crisis standards of care in a disaster situation. It also intends that by suggesting a uniform approach, consistency will develop across geographic and political boundaries so that this guidance will be useful in contributing to a single, national framework for responding to crisis in a fair, equitable, and transparent manner.

The committee appreciates the opportunity to begin to lay the foundation for this important two-phase project as well as the opportunity to help the nation prepare not only for the upcoming pandemic, but for all disaster scenarios where the health system may be stressed to its limits. We look forward to undertaking the second phase of this project, in which the committee will expand stakeholder and public engagement efforts, as well as update and expand the guidance based on input and feedback from individuals and groups involved in the development and implementation of crisis standards of care.

Lawrence O. Gostin, J.D., *Chair*
Dan Hanfling, M.D., *Vice Chair*
Committee on Guidance for Establishing
Standards of Care for Use in Disaster Situations

## BACKGROUND

The current influenza pandemic caused by the 2009 H1N1 virus underscores the immediate and critical need to prepare for a public health emergency in which thousands, tens of thousands, or even hundreds of thousands of people suddenly seek and require medical care in communities across the United States. Although this may occur over hours, days, or weeks, this overwhelming surge on the healthcare system will dramatically strain medical resources and could compromise the ability of healthcare professionals to adhere to normal treatment procedures and conventional standards of care. The Office of the Assistant Secretary for Preparedness and Response (ASPR), Department of Health and Human Services (HHS), charged the Institute of Medicine committee responsible for this study with the task of developing guidance to establish standards of care that should apply to disaster situations—both naturally occurring and manmade—under conditions in which resources are scarce (Box 1).

The Committee on Guidance for Establishing Standards of Care for Use in Disaster Situations brings together a broad spectrum of expertise, including state and local public health, emergency medicine and response, primary care, nursing, palliative care, ethics, the law, behavioral health, and risk communication (Appendix E). This letter report is not intended to obviate or substitute for extensive additional consideration and study of this complex issue, but is focused on articulating current concepts and preliminary guidance that can assist state and local public health officials, healthcare facilities, and professionals in the development of systematic and comprehensive policies and protocols for standards of care in disasters where resources are scarce. These policies and protocols must conform to rigorous standards of science, law, and ethics.

The committee focused its efforts on establishing a framework for the development and implementation of standards of care and associated triggers during disaster events. It was not responsible for establishing, creating, or defining what should be such crisis standards of care and associated triggers.

This guidance is intended to assist federal policy makers and state and local officials in the development of more extensive and nationally/regionally consistent crisis standards of care policies and protocols that are applicable to all disaster situations. The committee developed

---

**BOX 1**
**Statement of Task**

In response to a request from the Department of Health and Human Services' Office of the Assistant Secretary for Preparedness and Response (ASPR), the Institute of Medicine (IOM) will convene an ad hoc committee to conduct a two-phase activity on standards of care for use in disaster situations. The committee will focus attention on developing guidance to establish standards of care that should apply to disaster situations—both naturally occurring and manmade—where resources are scarce. Ethical principles will be incorporated into the standards.

Phase 1

An ad hoc committee of the IOM will conduct a study and issue a letter report to the ASPR by October 1, 2009. The letter report will provide guidance on standards of care for use in disaster situations. Specifically, the committee will:

- Develop preliminary framework guidance that identifies and describes the key elements that should be included in disaster standards of care protocols;
- Identify potential triggers that can be used by state and local public health officials to develop standards of care protocols that will assist healthcare providers;
- Develop a template matrix that can be used by state and local public health officials as a framework for developing specific guidance for healthcare providers to develop disaster standards of care;
- Consider roles and responsibilities of various stakeholders in the implementation of the guidance; and
- Consider mechanisms for integrating the views of the general public and healthcare providers in the development and implementation of the guidance.

The letter report will identify triggers that indicate a need to change from normal standards to disaster standards. Disaster standards will consider approaches to conserving, substituting, adapting. and doing without resources. The committee will not be responsible for establishing, creating, or defining standards of care.

The committee will also commission a paper to be delivered by September 1, 2009. This commissioned paper will provide background to the committee deliberations and will examine the key elements in existing state and local standards of care protocols and the impact of allocation schemes on disaster standards, and propose framework guidance for national disaster standards that can be applied to nH1N1 response for the coming fall flu season. In addition, the commissioned paper will explore issues related to the implementation of standards of care protocols, including legal considerations. The committee will base its recommendations on currently available policies, protocols, published literature, and other available guidance documents and evidence, as well as its expert judgment.

---

Phase 2
    Phase 2 of the project will prepare a report that will update the preliminary guidance developed in phase 1. The expanded guidance will be based on a series of stakeholder input activities. During this phase the committee will seek input and comment from individuals who used the guidance developed in phase I. In addition, the committee will organize and host a series of data-gathering activities focused on the provider community and the public (e.g., local civic organizations, leaders from faith-based groups, educators) that would allow an opportunity to provide comment on the guidance developed in phase 1. The expanded report will include considerations about triggers that apply to changes in the standards of care and approaches to conserving, substituting, adapting, and doing without resources. In addition, the committee will develop guidance that will include information for healthcare providers from primary care, home health, community health centers, and other provider communities not traditionally engaged.

two case studies that illustrate the application of the guidance and principles laid out in the report to two different scenarios (Appendix C). Recognizing the current attention and concern around the 2009 H1N1 pandemic, one scenario focuses on a gradual-onset pandemic flu, modeled around issues that may arise this upcoming flu season. The other scenario focuses on an earthquake and the particular issues that would arise during a no-notice event.

## 2009 H1N1 Influenza Pandemic and Other Public Health Emergencies and Disasters

    Although there is still significant uncertainty about the likely severity and extent of the 2009 H1N1 influenza outbreak in the fall, there is great concern that demand for healthcare services could increase dramatically, resulting in a severe strain on medical resources across the United States. Mexico reported the first case of the novel virus nH1N1 on April 12, 2009, and by June 11 the World Health Organization (WHO) raised its pandemic alert level to a full-blown pandemic. Within 9 weeks of the first reported cases, every WHO region reported cases, and now the virus has spanned the globe, affecting more than 170 countries (WHO, 2009b). The virus spread throughout most of the southern hemisphere during that region's winter influenza season, while continuing to circulate in the summer months in the northern hemisphere.
    In the United States, 9,079 hospitalizations and 593 deaths associated with 2009 H1N1 were reported to the Centers for Disease Control and Prevention (CDC) as of August 30, 2009 (CDC, 2009a). During the peak

U.S. influenza season, multiple viral strains may be circulating simultaneously—2009 H1N1 and seasonal influenza. Over the past few years, in anticipation of a severe pandemic of H5N1 ("bird flu") and other public health emergencies (e.g., bioterrorism), many states and healthcare institutions have been developing pandemic and other emergency preparedness plans that include enhancing healthcare system surge capacity to respond to catastrophic and mass casualty events. Government agencies and the healthcare system are now heavily preparing for the possibility of needing to implement their pandemic plans (or revised versions of them to reflect the current severity of the H1N1 pandemic) during the upcoming influenza season, even though at present 2009 H1N1 has not been highly pathogenic.

Although the 2009 H1N1 pandemic is currently receiving the highest attention in the medical and public health community, the nation also faces the possibility of many other potential public health emergencies and disasters that could severely strain medical resources. For example, the detonation of an improvised nuclear device in a large city would cause massive numbers of injured and dead (IOM, 2009a). Similarly, other disasters caused by terrorism or by natural causes, such as fires, floods, earthquakes, and hurricanes, have the potential to overwhelm the medical and public health systems.

## Scarce Resources, Demand for Healthcare Services, and Standards of Care

In preparation for response to any large-scale disaster or public health emergency, healthcare facilities are developing surge plans that include efforts to increase and maximize use of available resources, as well as to manage demand for healthcare services. Facilities can use resource-sharing agreements (e.g., mutual aid agreements) and other mechanisms that enable full use of the community's resources, which should include the regional resources and capabilities of the health systems of the Veterans Administration, the Department of Defense (DoD), and Indian Health Services. Communities may also request resource support from state and federal disaster supply caches, including those of the Strategic National Stockpile. However, in the setting of an influenza pandemic, where the shortage of resources is likely to occur on a national scale, the availability of such supplementary support is much less certain. Beyond preparedness stocking, facilities can also implement a variety of strategies that permit conservation, reuse, adaptation, and substitution for certain resources, doing so in a way that minimizes the impact on clinical care (Rubinson et al., 2008b; Rubinson et al., 2008a; Minnesota Department of Health, August 2008). To manage demand, surge plans may also include the use of an alternate care system that allows for the delivery of healthcare services along a stratified spectrum which includes home health care, community-based care, and the use of alternate care facilities (Hick et al., 2004; Kaji et al., 2006; Barbisch and Koenig, 2006; Davis et al., 2005; Hanfling, 2006; California Department of Public Health, 2008; Kelen et al., 2009).

However, these measures may not always be sufficient, especially in a wide-reaching public health emergency or disaster in which resources are simultaneously strained in communities across the nation. Faced with severe shortages of equipment, supplies, and pharmaceuticals, an insufficient number of qualified healthcare providers, overwhelming demand for services, and a lack of suitable space, healthcare practitioners will have to make difficult decisions about how to allocate these limited resources if contingency plans do not accommodate incident demands. Under these circumstances, it may be impossible to provide care according to the conventional standards of care used in non-disaster situations, and, under the most extreme circumstances, it may not even be possible to provide the most basic life-sustaining interventions to all patients who need them. The impact of these circumstances will likely carry a tremendous social cost on the healthcare workforce and the nation as a whole.

An important consideration regarding the framework for the implementation of crisis standards of care in a disaster includes the recognition that it will never be an "all or none" situation. Disasters will have varying impacts on communities, based on many different variables that might affect the delivery of health care during such events. Response to a surge in demand for healthcare services will likely fall along a continuum ranging from "conventional" to "contingency" and "crisis" surge responses (Hick et al., 2009).

Conventional patient care uses usual resources to deliver health and medical care that conforms to the expected standards of care of the community. The delivery of care in the setting of contingency surge response seeks to provide patient care that remains *functionally equivalent* to conventional care. Contingency care adapts available patient care spaces, staff, and supplies as part of the response to a surge in demand for services. Although this may introduce minor risk to the patient compared to usual care (e.g., substituting less familiar medications for those in short supply, thereby potentially leading to medication dosage error), the overall delivery of care remains mostly consistent with community standards. Crisis care, however, occurs under conditions in which usual safeguards are no longer possible. Crisis care is provided when available resources are insufficient to meet usual care standards, thus providing a transition point to implementing *crisis standards of care.* Note that in an important ethical sense, entering a crisis standard of care mode is not optional – it is a forced choice, based on the emerging situation. Under such circumstances, failing to make substantive adjustments to care op-erations – i.e., not to adopt crisis standards of care – is very likely to re-sult in greater death, injury or illness. The goal for the health system is to increase the ability to stay in conventional and contingency categories through preparedness and anticipation of resource needs prior to serious shortages, and to return as quickly as possible from crisis back across the continuum to conventional care.

Recognizing that such a spectrum exists may help communities iden-tify where they are along this continuum, provide a uniform and consis-tent way to evaluate and report surge conditions, and illustrate the spectrum of adaptations required to address the situation.

## State and Local Policies and Protocols

The issue of crisis standards of care for use in disaster situations in-volving scarce resources arose largely since 2004, when the Agency for Healthcare Research and Quality (AHRQ) and the ASPR within HHS convened a meeting of experts. Drawn from the fields of bioethics, emergency medicine, emergency management, health administration, law and policy, and public health, experts engaged in groundbreaking discussions and confronted these issues directly. Their deliberations led to a report, *Altered Standards of Care in Mass Casualty Events* (AHRQ, 2005b), which laid out major concerns and areas that require considera-tion and recommended next steps for future action. A subsequent report, *Mass Medical Care with Scarce Resources: A Community Planning Guide*, laid down the framework for much of the current planning efforts (Phillips and Knebel, 2007).

Since the release of the 2005 AHRQ report, many federal, state, and local efforts to develop protocols for the allocation of scarce resources and for standards of care have occurred. Nevertheless, a recent report on state preparedness by the U.S. Government Accountability Office (GAO) and a recent review of HHS's Hospital Preparedness Program by the Center for Biosecurity of UPMC concluded that among the key components of medical surge planning, "standards of care during a mass casualty event" remained in need of significant additional attention and planning (GAO, June 2008; Toner et al., 2009). Areas of particular concern cited were the need for states to develop protocols for implementing standards of care in disaster situations and the need to achieve a higher level of consistency across neighboring jurisdictions.

Federal policy makers and state and local officials, in consultation with stakeholders from the private healthcare sector, could use the results of this committee's work to inform the development of more extensive and nationally/regionally consistent standards of care policies and protocols.

## METHODS

To conduct this expert assessment and develop guidance for establishing standards of care for use in disasters, the committee met from September 1 to 4, 2009. The meeting included a day-long public workshop (see Appendix D). The purpose of the workshop was to hear from the public and experts with a wide breadth of experience and perspectives on this topic. In addition, the committee also heard from relevant stakeholder organizations, including federal agencies and representatives from key components of the public health system and healthcare system, to inform the committee about relevant ongoing and planned initiatives. Finally, the committee commissioned a white paper by Dr. Jeffrey Dichter and Dr. Michael Christian that provided a broad overview of many of the currently available standards of care protocols. Throughout the report terms such as "crisis standards of care" or "triage team" have been used. Recognizing potential confusion, the committee developed a glossary to define the report's key terms (Appendix B).

Additional background and context for the committee's work was provided by a series of four regional meetings held in the spring of 2009 by the Institute of Medicine's Forum on Medical and Public Health Preparedness for Catastrophic Events. These regional meetings on Standards of Care During Mass Casualty Events were designed to describe and demonstrate the current regional, state, and local efforts to establish disaster standards of care policies, and to improve regional efforts by facilitating dialogue and coordination among neighboring jurisdictions.

During these meetings, many state and local officials identified the need for national guidance on standards of care for disaster situations as a crucial area for improving the nation's preparedness (IOM, 2009c). The committee performed a limited literature review that included more than 200 references. In addition, the committee specifically reviewed a number of available standards of care protocols from states and other government agencies (Veterans Health Administration or VHA; the states of California, Colorado, Massachusetts, Minnesota, New York, Utah, Virginia, and Washington; and the Canadian province of Ontario).

This letter report is based on the committee's expert judgment and assessment of the currently available policies and protocols, published literature and other available guidance documents and evidence, and the workshop presentations and discussions. The compressed schedule limited the scope of work presented here, but most importantly, it greatly limited the committee's ability to perform an extensive engagement with community and provider stakeholders. However, phase 2 will allow the committee to carry out a more deliberative project that will specifically include expanded stakeholder and public engagement efforts. It will also provide an opportunity to update and expand the crisis standards of care guidance based on input and feedback from individuals involved in the development and implementation of crisis standards of care.

## CRISIS STANDARDS OF CARE: THE VISION

The U.S. health system affords many Americans a high quality of health care. Existing levels of health care in routine situations in the United States are unlikely to be available in times of a mass disaster involving scarce resources. Therefore, the United States must continue to plan for a catastrophic public health event that will cause grave injury, disease, or death to potentially thousands or tens or hundreds of thousands in a city, region, or entire nation. Public health emergencies such as a novel infectious disease (e.g., 2009 H1N1 or severe acute respiratory syndrome [SARS]), an intentional release of a biological agent (e.g., anthrax or smallpox), or a weather or climatic event (e.g., hurricane or tornado) highlight the ever-changing threats posed by naturally occurring and intentional threats to the public's health.

To plan for a catastrophic event, the nation needs to prepare conscientiously and systematically to ensure that (1) the response offers the best care possible given the resources at hand; (2) decisions are fair and transparent; (3) policies and protocols within and across states are consistent; and (4) citizens and stakeholders are included and heard. Laws and the legal environment must support response efforts and create incentives for healthcare practitioners to care for affected populations. Although the usual high quality of health services cannot be assured during a catastrophic event, the nation must do all it can to gain the trust of the public by responding fairly and effectively, particularly for vulnerable persons (Gostin and Powers, 2006).

The committee was tasked to develop national framework guidance on the key elements that should be included in standards of care protocols for disaster situations. Ethical goals in medical care do not change, including during disasters – health care professionals are obligated always to provide the best care they can under given circumstances. The committee defines the optimal level of health and medical care that can be delivered during a catastrophic event as *crisis standards of care*.

> Crisis standards of care: A substantial change in usual healthcare operations and the level of care it is possible to deliver, which is made necessary by a pervasive (e.g., pandemic influenza) or catastrophic (e.g., earthquake, hurricane) disaster. This change in the level of care delivered is justified by specific circumstances and is formally declared by a state government, in recognition that crisis operations will be in effect for a sustained period. The formal declaration that crisis standards of care are in operation enables specific legal/regulatory powers and protections for healthcare providers in the necessary tasks of allocating and using scarce medical resources and implementing alternate care facility operations.

To ensure that the best care possible is provided to patients in a catastrophic event, the nation needs robust and carefully-developed guidance for the public, healthcare professionals and institutions, and governmental entities at all levels. The committee sets forth the following vision for crisis standards of care:

- *Fairness*—standards that are, to the highest degree possible, recognized as fair by all those affected by them – including the members of affected communities, practitioners, and provider organizations, evidence based and responsive to specific needs of individuals and the population focused on a duty of compassion and care, a duty to steward resources, and a goal of maintaining the trust of patients and the community

- *Equitable processes*—processes and procedures for ensuring that decisions and implementation of standards are made equitably
  - *Transparency*—in design and decision making
  - *Consistency*—in application across populations and among individuals regardless of their human condition (e.g., race, age, disability, ethnicity, ability to pay, socioeconomic status, preexisting health conditions, social worth, perceived obstacles to treatment, past use of resources)
  - *Proportionality*—public and individual requirements must be commensurate with the scale of the emergency and degree of scarce resources
  - *Accountability*—of individuals deciding and implementing standards, and of governments for ensuring appropriate protections and just allocation of available resources
- *Community and provider engagement, education, and communication*—active collaboration with the public and stakeholders for their input is essential through formalized processes
- *The rule of law*
  - *Authority*—to empower necessary and appropriate actions and interventions in response to emergencies
  - *Environment*—to facilitate implementation through laws that support standards and create appropriate incentives

### Five Key Elements of Crisis Standards of Care Protocols

Based on a review of a number of standards of care protocols (California Department of Public Health, 2008; Virginia Department of Health, 2008; Powell et al., 2008; Colorado Department of Public Health and Environment, 2009; Minnesota Department of Health, 2008; The Commonwealth of Massachusetts Department of Public Health, May 2007; Levin et al., 2009; The Utah Hospitals and Health Systems Association, 2009; Ontario Ministry of Health and Long-Term Care, 2008; VHA, 2008, 2009; Washington State Department of Health's Altered Standards of Care Workgroup, October 2008), published literature, and discussion at the workshop, the committee identified and defined five key elements that should be included in all crisis standards-of care-protocols. These five key elements each have several associated components (Table 1), which will be described in greater detail throughout the remainder of this report. To ensure that crisis standards of care protocols enable a response that is ethical, legal, and consistent within and across state borders, states in partnership with localities should ensure that they address, at a minimum, each of these key elements and corresponding components.

> **Recommendation 1: <u>Develop Consistent State Crisis Standards of Care Protocols with Five Key Elements</u>**
> **State departments of health, and other relevant state agencies, in partnership with localities should ensure that crisis standards of care protocols include five key elements—and associated components—detailed in this report:**
>
> - **A strong ethical grounding;**
> - **Integrated and ongoing community and provider engagement, education, and communication;**
> - **Assurances regarding legal authority and environment;**
> - **Clear indicators, triggers, and lines of responsibility; and**
> - **Evidence-based clinical processes and operations.**

**TABLE 1** Five Key Elements of Crisis Standards of Care Protocols and Associated Components

| Key Elements of Crisis Standards of Care Protocols | Components |
| --- | --- |
| Ethical considerations | o  Fairness<br>o  Duty to care<br>o  Duty to steward resources<br>o  Transparency<br>o  Consistency<br>o  Proportionality<br>o  Accountability |
| Community and provider engagement, education, and communication | o  Community stakeholder identification with delineation of roles and involvement with attention to vulnerable populations<br>o  Community trust and assurance of fairness and transparency in processes developed<br>o  Community cultural values and boundaries<br>o  Continuum of community education and trust building<br>o  Crisis risk communication strategies and situational awareness<br>o  Continuum of resilience building and mental health triage<br>o  Palliative care education for stakeholders |
| Legal authority and environment | o  Medical and legal standards of care<br>o  Scope of practice for healthcare professionals<br>o  Mutual aid agreements to facilitate resource allocation<br>o  Federal, state, and local declarations of:<br>    o  Emergency<br>    o  Disaster<br>    o  Public health emergency<br>o  Special emergency protections (e.g., PREP Act, Section 1135 waivers of sanctions under EMTALA and HIPAA Privacy Rule)<br>o  Licensing and credentialing<br>o  Medical malpractice |

| Key Elements of Crisis Standards of Care Protocols | Components |
| --- | --- |
| | o   Liability risks (civil, criminal, Constitutional) |
| | o   Statutory, regulatory, and common-law liability protections |
| Indicators and triggers | Indicators for assessment and potential management |
| | o   Situational awareness (local/regional, state, national) |
| | o   Event specific |
| |     o   Illness and injury—incidence and severity |
| |     o   Disruption of social and community functioning |
| |     o   Resource availability |
| | Triggers for action |
| | o   Critical infrastructure disruption |
| | o   Failure of "contingency" surge capacity (resource-sparing strategies overwhelmed) |
| |     o   Human resource/staffing availability |
| |     o   Material resource availability |
| |     o   Patient care space availability |
| Clinical process and operations | Local/regional and state government processes to include: |
| | o   State-level "disaster medical advisory committee" and local "Clinical care committees" and "triage teams." |
| | o   Resource-sparing strategies |
| | o   Incident management (NIMS/HICS) principles |
| | o   Intrastate and interstate regional consistencies in the application of crisis standards of care |
| | o   Coordination of resource management |
| | o   Specific attention to vulnerable populations and those with medical special needs |
| | o   Communications strategies |

| Key Elements of Crisis Standards of Care Protocols | Components |
|---|---|
| | o  Coordination extends through all elements of the health system, including public health, emergency medical services, long-term care, primary care, and home care |
| | Clinical operations based on crisis surge response plan: <br> o  Decision support tool to triage life-sustaining interventions <br> o  Palliative care principles <br> o  Mental health needs and promotion of resilience |

## DEVELOPING CRISIS STANDARDS OF CARE PROTOCOLS: A STATE PUBLIC HEALTH AUTHORITY PROCESS

State authorities have the political and constitutional mandate to prepare for and coordinate the response to disaster situations throughout their state jurisdictions. Consequently, states in partnership with localities have the responsibility for developing crisis standards of care protocols for use in disaster situations that result in severely limited healthcare resources. In most states, the state department of health holds this responsibility. Some states have well-defined processes for establishing their protocols, but many others are still in development. This report contains guidance to assist state public health authorities in developing these crisis standards of care in partnership with their regional and local public health authorities, including the key elements that should be included in the crisis standards of care protocols and criteria for determining when crisis standards of care should be implemented.

Although the state authority has the responsibility to establish, and ultimately determine, when to implement crisis standards of care, stakeholders should be important partners in this process, including healthcare professionals and institutions, public health and emergency management agencies, and state residents. The following is a framework for the development of crisis standards of care with a series of action steps for the state authority. This framework is based on the guidance laid out in this report and the experience of several states that have already developed, or started developing, protocols.

1. **Outline Ethical Considerations:** Convene a "Guideline Development Working Group" of appropriate stakeholders to establish ethical principles that will serve as the basis for the crisis standards of care. The group should include (but is not limited to) representatives of regional and local health authorities, healthcare providers and representatives from professional associations, ethicists, patient advocates, public health and healthcare attorneys, community-based organizations, and members of the faith community. The ethics section in this report provides a comprehensive basis for these deliberations. Some states have also found it useful to develop scenarios to assist in recognizing and understanding the difficult decisions that will confront healthcare providers when resources are inadequate (New Jersey Hospital Association, 2008; Massachusetts Department of Public Health and Center for Public Health Preparedness, 2006).

2. **Review Legal Authority for Implementation of Crisis Standards of Care:** Review existing legal authority for the implementation of crisis standards of care and address legal issues related to the successful implementation of these standards, such as liability protections or temporary changes in licensure or certification status or scope of practice. Revise and reform laws (statutory, regulatory) or policies as necessary (California Department of Public Health, 2008). These and other considerations are carefully set out later in the report.

3. **Develop Guidance for Provision of Medical Care Under State Crisis Standards of Care:** Establish an "Advisory Committee," which can include members of the Guideline Development Working Group (see above composition), but should also be expanded to include comprehensive representation from healthcare practitioners and professional associations in relevant specialties, including but not limited to nurses, physicians, emergency medical technicians, a range of specialists from pediatrics to geriatrics, mental health, palliative care, healthcare facilities, and other relevant entities such as the American Red Cross. Although this committee's deliberations will focus on complex medical issues, ethicists and public safety specialists should also be included in

the committee to ensure that considerations from these disciplines are integrated into the protocols. Crisis standards of care should be consistent with the ethical elements developed by the Guideline Development Working Group. This committee will find a comprehensive set of materials to inform its deliberations in the "Indicators and Triggers" and "Clinical Process and Operations" sections of this report. Note that this Advisory Committee is a planning group for specific crisis standards of care situations. The Committee members' roles during a disaster should also be defined (see #5).

4. **Conduct a Public Stakeholder Engagement Process:** Although representatives of various healthcare and other interested professional groups and the public have been involved in drafting the ethical principles and crisis standards of care, a robust engagement process is also necessary to provide an opportunity for review and comment by the provider and public community at large. Particular attention should be paid to outreach to and input from vulnerable populations, including those with medical special needs. At these meetings, discussion should include an explanation of the need for crisis standards of care, the process for development of these standards, when and how crisis standards of care would be implemented, and an opportunity for those in attendance to comment on the drafts. Although these steps are an integral component of establishing standards of care protocols, few authorities have actively engaged in these efforts. Guidance on this process is provided in the "Community and Provider Engagement" section. In addition, the state of New York and Seattle and King County both have integrated these into their protocol development processes (Powell et al., 2008; Li-Vollmer, 2009).

Following the public engagement process, the ethical elements and crisis standards of care can be finalized, incorporating, as appropriate, changes based on comments received. Communication and education on crisis standards of care with healthcare professionals and institutions and the public should continue as part of the general approach to public health emergency preparedness.

5. **Establish a Medical Disaster Advisory Committee:** During a disaster, this committee will provide ongoing advice to the state authority regarding changes to the situation and potential corresponding changes in the implementation of crisis standards of care. The Advisory Committee (see #3) responsible for developing the crisis standards of care, or a subcommittee of those members, with additional members having the requisite expertise to perform this function for the specific disaster, can serve in this capacity. This group may be asked to provide input on a wider range of medical care issues during a disaster for which consistent state policy is required and thus should be able to call on technical medical expertise from a variety of areas according to the event specifics (critical care, emergency medical services, emergency medicine, toxicology, infectious disease, trauma/burn care, radiation injury, etc.). The composition of the committee should include individuals informed by real life experience who have had personal responsibility for coordinating healthcare system response and mitigation efforts to large-scale disaster events, with practical know how, and experience and understanding of the 'system' of response. Members should understand their roles and responsibilities and be available to the state during an event in person or at least via phone. Because providers may have other event-related obligations, this group should have several persons listed in each area of expertise. In addition, as will be described in more detail later in the report, during a disaster the Medical Disaster Advisory Committee will work closely at a local level with "clinical care committees" and "triage teams."

Several states and localities have begun to develop scarce resource allocation protocols; however, few have provided guidelines for decision tools that will be needed during an incident (California Department of Public Health, 2008; Virginia Department of Health, 2008; Powell et al., 2008; Colorado Department of Public Health and Environment, 2009; The Commonwealth of Massachusetts Department of Public Health, May 2007; Levin et al., 2009; Minnesota Department of Health, 2008; The Utah Hospitals and Health Systems Association, 2009; Washington State Department of Health's Altered Standards of Care Workgroup, October 2008; Houston/Harris County Committee, 2007). Ontario has also developed protocols that include additional consideration for crisis standards of care for patients with cancer or chronic renal disease/acute renal injury, as well as in regard to blood services and long-term care (Ontario Ministry of Health and Long-term Care, 2008). Local communities have also engaged in developing such ethical frameworks for their respective localities, including the Houston/Harris County area, which has developed local community guidance for medical standards of care around pandemic influenza planning based on ethical deliberations and community input (Houston/Harris County Committee, 2007). In addition, the VHA has developed a protocol for allocation of scarce life-saving resources in the VHA during an influenza pandemic, along with an ethical framework that underlies the protocol (VHA, 2008, 2009). The state health departments in New York and California as well as the VHA have begun to develop guidance for allocation of ventilators. These protocols form the basis of much of this committee's deliberations and could serve as useful models for those states that are just beginning the process of developing crisis standards of care protocols. To ensure consistent implementation, states should ensure that protocol development is in accordance with the guidance and key elements outlined in this report, but existing state protocols could be used to avoid unnecessary duplication of effort and as a model for developing and implementing those key elements at the appropriate level of detail.

In recognition of the extensive work already undertaken by many states, and the need for other states to develop their own processes and protocols, the committee supports the GAO's and UPMC's Center for Biosecurity recommendations for a clearinghouse that should be developed and housed by the HHS (GAO, 2008; Toner et al., 2009). This "clearinghouse," or other easily accessed electronic repository, should include model standards of care protocols developed by the states, localities, and other groups, relevant peer-reviewed literature, and model tools that could be integrated into planning and implementation strategies.

## ETHICAL FRAMEWORK

An ethical framework serves as the bedrock for public policy. In developing ethically sound policies for providing health care in disasters, the committee urges policy makers and communities to keep in mind current and past inequities in the allocation of healthcare resources and in healthcare outcomes and try to avoid these in future events through careful policy design. Among the lessons of Hurricane Katrina and other large-scale disasters is that those communities that are most vulnerable before a disaster are likely the most vulnerable during a disaster. Ethically and clinically sound planning will aim to secure equitable allocation of resources and fair protections for vulnerable groups as compared to the general population.

During disasters, healthcare professionals may question whether they can maintain core professional values and behaviors. They wonder if it is possible to uphold core professional values and behaviors in the context of disaster. Is a nurse who provides critical care to 10 patients in a disaster acting unethically, as could be the case under ordinary circumstances? Professionals may ask which choices and standards might properly shift during a disaster, and when core ethical values draw a bright line that separates behaviors that are acceptable from those that are unacceptable. A useful disaster policy will help these persons judge how to act as good professionals even in emergency circumstances.

## Ethical Norms

There are many principles that can contribute to an ethical framework. Various authors have articulated principles for public health and disaster ethics (Childress et al., 2002; University of Toronto Joint Centre for Bioethics Pandemic Influenza Working Group, November 2005). We focus here on a limited set of essential elements that reflect both core substantive ethical values and processes, and that can serve as a model or a starting point for local deliberations. Ethical values include the concept of fairness and the professional duties to care and to steward resources. Ethical process elements include transparency, consistency, proportionality, and accountability. Tensions often arise between different ethical principles. Duties to care for individuals and to steward resources may come into conflict, for example. The Guideline Development Working Group should determine how best to weigh competing demands given local values, priorities and available resources.

### *Fairness*

The overarching ethical goal in developing crisis standards of care protocols is for them to be recognized as fair by all affected parties — even including those who might later be disadvantaged by the protocols. All subsequent ethical considerations reflect an effort to achieve such fairness. Fair crisis standards of care protocols will help communities and professionals act using just principles under harsh circumstances. Policy makers must seek to eliminate ways in which irrelevant factors such as class, race, ethnicity, neighborhood, or personal connections shift the burden of disaster toward vulnerable groups. By the same token, if particular groups receive favorable treatment, for instance in access to vaccines, this priority should stem from relevant factors (e.g., greater exposure or vulnerability) and promote important community goals (CDC, 2009c). Policies should reflect awareness of existing disparities in access to care, take account of the needs of the most vulnerable, and support the equitable and just distribution of scarce goods and resources.

Allocation choices based on evidence are one way to reflect the principle of fairness. This report will reference various disaster allocation schemes that rely on measurable and objective clinical parameters to help clinicians make difficult decisions in ways that are clear, consistent, and rational. Under duress, professionals may not be able to create fair allocation schemes in real-time. Disaster planning must include advance ethical guidance. Factors such as do-not-resuscitate (DNR) status have on occasion been considered in allocation schemes. However, DNR orders reflect individual preferences and foresight to establish advance directives more than an accurate estimate of survival. Accordingly, DNR orders are not useful parameters for considering the allocation of scarce resources.

### Duty to Care

The primary duty of a health care professional is to the patient in need of medical care. This duty holds true during disasters, including when providing care entails some risk to the clinician (AMA, 2004). Because of this strong and deep obligation, health professionals are educated primarily to care for individuals and less so for populations, although all health professionals also do have important public health obligations (Wynia, 2005). Even in crisis situations, however, clinicians cannot relinquish their obligations to individuals without sacrificing core professional values. The covenant between professional and patient gains rather than loses value in a public health disaster, when members of the community are justifiably frightened and numerous institutions and support systems face great strain. Recognizing that scarce resources may restrict treatment choices, clinicians must not abandon, and patients should not fear abandonment, when an ethical framework informs healthcare disaster policy.

Ethics elements of disaster policies should support the professional's duty to care. For instance, policies that outline role sequestration, separating those with triage responsibilities from those providing direct care, help preserve the professional integrity of healthcare workers. Those providing direct care can work to improve the health status of their individual patients and will not simultaneously be expected to make decisions that limit care.

While professionals have a duty to care for patients, healthcare institutions have a reciprocal duty to support healthcare workers (The Pandemic Influenza Ethics Initiative, 2009). Personal protective equipment, engineering controls, and a variety of mechanisms to reduce the risk of infection demonstrate institutional obligations to protect workers who face risks in providing care (IOM, 2009b). Various types of disasters might call for other or additional protections to safeguard healthcare workers who face risks, including mental health risks, as they provide care to the community.

*Duty to Steward Resources*

Healthcare institutions and public health officials also have a duty to steward scarce resources, reflecting the utilitarian goal of saving the greatest possible number of lives. Professionals must balance this duty to the community against that to the individual patient. Though clinicians face this dilemma under ordinary circumstances, the level of scarcity in a public health disaster exacerbates this tension. As scarcity increases, accommodating the two competing duties of care and stewardship will require more difficult choices (Pesik et al., 2001).

There is no uniform answer about how to weigh such competing values, especially when under the duress of time constraints, emotional and physical stress, and while assimilating fluctuating or rapidly emerging new information. Addressing this balancing act under very difficult conditions, with the goal of making decisions that will be recognized as fair under the circumstances, makes it critical to establish ethical *processes* for decision-making.

# Ethical Process

*Transparency*

Public entities charged with protecting communities during disasters have profound responsibilities. They are called on to plan for foreseeable disasters. They must draw on the best available research, collect and develop expert opinion, and draw attention to gaps in knowledge and resources needed to protect the community. But ethically sound disaster policies require more than technical expertise. These policies must reflect specific values in choices about contested issues, such as priority setting for access to scarce resources and restrictions on individual choice. A public engagement process is crucial for drafting ethical policies that reflect the communities' values and deserve its trust. However, though various scholars and public entities are currently in the midst of projects that engage the public, the goal of effective community participation in disaster policy development and evaluation is insufficiently realized at this time (CDC, 2009c; Li-Vollmer, 2009; Bernier, 2009; Bernier and Marcuse, December 2005). Given that a more severe influenza pandemic may emerge before the completion of a robust process of public engagement, officials must strive to communicate clearly those plans currently in place, and may also need to rely on real-time communication with communities and after-the-fact review.

A truly inclusive process will not rely only on input from professional groups and other organized stakeholders, but will also incorporate the views of those who are less well represented in the political process, but who may be greatly affected by policy choices. Children and their parents, older adults, persons with disabilities, and racially and ethnically diverse communities are more likely to feel keenly the impact of different choices in priority setting. Policies should reflect their values no less than those of other sectors of society. Enlisting the public to discuss a future disaster when current stressors overwhelm many will prove challenging, but is nonetheless required. An ethical process will likely be iterative, characterized by responsible planning, transparency in underlying values and priorities, robust efforts toward public engagement, response to public comment, commitment to ongoing revision of policy based on dialogue and data, and accountability for support and implementation.

Values that drive policy should be explicitly stated so communities can articulate, examine, affirm or reject, and modify proposed choices.

Transparency also implies candor in communication about disasters, from clinicians to patients and throughout all levels of the healthcare system. Limitation of choice for both patients and providers is a reality of disaster and will affect many aspects of healthcare delivery. Professionals and patients will have fewer treatment options. Evidence-based criteria, rather than patient preference or clinical judgment, will determine access to the most limited resources. Though patient autonomy is reduced by the circumstances of disaster, patients still deserve clear information about available choices, respect for preferences within resource constraints, and empathic acknowledgment of the sometimes dire consequences of resource limitation.

*Consistency*

Consistency in treating like groups alike is one way of promoting fairness. The public may find that scarce resources have not been allocated fairly if patients at different hospitals in the same affected area receive vastly different levels of care. Consistent policies may also help eliminate unfair local efforts to discriminate against vulnerable groups on the basis of factors such as race or disability. However, efforts to keep policies consistent across institutions or geographic regions may limit local flexibility in implementing guidance. The capacity for local communities to reflect their values in allocating scarce resources stands in tension with the goal of promoting consistency. Flexibility is necessary, but requires careful deliberation and documentation where local practices do not follow common guidance.

*Proportionality*

Disaster policies will include aspects that are burdensome to individuals and professionals. Burdens such as social distancing, school closures, or even quarantine should be necessary and commensurate with the scale of the public health disaster. Those restrictions imposed must serve important public needs, such as the need to limit spread of an infectious agent, and must be appropriately limited in time and scale according to the scope and severity of the disaster.

*Accountability*

Effective disaster planning will require individuals at all levels of the healthcare system to accept and act upon appropriate responsibilities. As part of their duties to care and to steward scarce resources, individual clinicians are responsible for a good faith effort toward education in important disaster-related concepts and knowledge of local planning efforts (AMA, 2004). Local facilities are accountable for disaster policies. Government entities are accountable to their communities to plan and implement policies related to disasters, and members of the community must know which entities take responsibility for various elements of disaster policies. For instance, practitioners concerned about the provision of personal protective equipment should know which entity is accountable for that domain and to whom they should address concerns. All decision-makers should be accountable for a reasonable level of situational awareness and for incorporating evidence into decision-making, including revising decisions as new data emerge. Like transparency, consistency and proportionality, accountability before, during and after a disaster is a key ingredient in building and maintaining trust.

## Applying the Ethics Framework: Ventilator Allocation

The ethics framework described above serves as a guide in developing disaster policies. We examine here the hard choices involving the allocation of ventilators, beginning at the systems level and then for individual patients. Ventilators, of course, are only one of many elements that may sustain the life of a critically ill patient. Appropriate surge planning will balance the need to stockpile a range of critical resources, as well as staff and space to provide treatment. However, ventilator allocation serves as a useful example of decision making under conditions of scarcity for several reasons. Ventilators are large and expensive; facilities cannot provide more than a certain number of ventilators, even when all surge resources are in play. Furthermore, ventilators require trained staff to operate them and availability of necessary medications, and thus depend on the additional scarce resources of personnel and drugs. In an influenza pandemic, severe respiratory illness will also increase the need for and scarcity of ventilators. Finally, a ventilator is a discrete resource that cannot be titrated or shared effectively, and whose absence is highly likely to result in death.

First, we will examine ventilator allocation as applied to a specific group. A number of disaster policies address the controversial issue of how chronically ventilator-dependent patients figure in triage schemes. The VHA provides a thoughtful review of this problem, contrasting two different policy choices (The Pandemic Influenza Ethics Initiative, 2009). It notes that the New York State Task Force on Life & the Law argued for exempting patients in long-term care facilities from ventilator triage protocols because extubation of stable chronic care patients would force clinicians in long-term care facilities into an unacceptable reversal of their caring role (NYSDOH/NYS Task Force on Life & the Law, 2007). Moreover, the reallocation of ventilators from chronic care patients would impose an unfair burden on the disabled, in part based on subjective quality-of-life judgments rather than on more objective estimates of survival. The Task Force found that patients in chronic care facilities should maintain access to ventilators while in those facilities. However, if transferred to an acute care facility, such patients should enter the triage system. In contrast, the World Health Organization concluded that chronic care patients should be included with all other patients in triage protocols, holding that all must share the sacrifice involved in triage equally (WHO, 2006). The VHA found that viable ethical arguments could support either position. The VHA chose to exclude from triage protocols those patients chronically supported by ventilators and living in long-term care facilities or at home, arguing that this choice represented the best available balance between the duty to care and to exercise stewardship of scarce resources.

Regarding ventilator allocation as applied to individual patients and healthcare professionals, disaster plans must minimize the need for such painful choices by requiring that all possible steps to augment and substitute for scarce resources precede any reallocation of scarce resources. Yet, if need sufficiently overwhelms resources, not all patients who might benefit from critical care resources can receive them.

Alternative allocation criteria could proceed on a first-come, first-served basis or through a lottery system, but either of these systems would result in excess mortality because some patients who receive ventilator treatment will die, and others who might have survived will die without it. Thus, this model of allocation would not uphold the duty to steward resources wisely and save the greatest possible number of lives. Several disaster policies reviewed by this committee require the use of evidence-based tools to assess the likelihood of benefit from critical care resources, and the reallocation of such resources under conditions of extreme scarcity to patients with the greatest likelihood of benefit when a clear and substantial difference in prognosis exists. These policies comport with an ethical framework that stewards resources and saves the greatest number of lives. It is important that these policies be explained, discussed, and considered by states developing crisis standards of care.

Many clinicians are justifiably troubled by the prospect of discontinuing life-sustaining treatment from a patient in a disaster, even though the purpose is to save lives. Clinicians at the bedside working under extreme circumstances deserve clarity, and without it they may be reluctant to implement a disaster standards of care protocol. Certainly, critical care physicians may discontinue life-prolonging treatment in response to a patient's request. The disaster context is agonizing because treatment could be withdrawn without or against the patient's expressed wishes. Ventilator withdrawal also requires an order not to resuscitate because resuscitation efforts require the use of ventilators. Outside of crisis situations, these orders typically require consent of patients or their surrogate decision makers, but disaster triage protocols may permit doctors to initiate such orders when life-sustaining treatment is reallocated.

What a disaster triage policy based on the duty to steward resources would do is effectively override individual patient preferences and instead supply resources based on evidence-based assessments of the benefit of the treatment relative to its scarcity. Thus, treatment offered in circumstances of a disaster should be understood as provisional—if the intervention is unsuccessful, it may be discontinued in order to provide the best possible care to as many as possible.

When resource scarcity reaches catastrophic levels, clinicians are ethically justified in using those resources to sustain life and well-being to the greatest extent possible. In the case of discontinuing life-sustaining treatment such as a ventilator, clinicians look to all ethical elements of the framework, starting with the principle of fairness. This hard choice stems from adherence to the duties to provide care and steward resources and follows guidance for ethical processes, including transparency, consistency, proportionality, and accountability.

Despite removing a vital treatment, a clinician must continue to provide compassionate care. In stewarding resources, palliative care will be prioritized to those critically ill patients who do not meet allocation criteria for scarce resources.

Transparency regarding limited resources forms a critical part of communication even before, but certainly during, a patient's hospital admission. Clinicians and facilities need to inform patients and families of the time-limited nature of trials of ventilator therapy and other scarce resources. Consistency in applying evidence-based triage tools helps guarantee fairness in access to resources, and provides professionals a clear rationale for triage decisions. Proportionality requires that this drastic infringement on the autonomous choice of patients or the professional judgment of clinicians is not invoked unless all other reasonable surge strategies have been implemented. Finally, accountability demands that professionals follow triage guidelines for assigning scarce resources and can support their decisions based on good-faith efforts to adhere to disaster policies. Professionals reasonably insist that adequate legal protection must accompany this shift from ordinary to crisis standards of care.

Crisis standards permit clinicians to allocate scarce resources so as to provide necessary and available treatments to patients most likely to benefit. Crisis standards do not permit clinicians to simply ignore professional norms and act without ethical standards or accountability. Crisis standards justify limiting access to scarce treatments, but neither the law nor ethics support the intentional hastening of death, even in a crisis.

> **Recommendation 2: Adhere to Ethical Norms in Crisis Standards of Care**
> **When crisis standards of care prevail, as when ordinary standards are in effect, healthcare practitioners must adhere to ethical norms. Conditions of overwhelming scarcity limit autonomous choices for both patients and practitioners regarding the allocation of scarce healthcare resources, but do not permit actions that violate ethical norms.**

## COMMUNITY AND PROVIDER ENGAGEMENT, EDUCATION, AND COMMUNICATION

Meaningful community engagement efforts for the general public, community leaders, and healthcare professionals are critical for the successful development, dissemination, and implementation of crisis standards of care. Community engagement is defined "as structured dialogue, joint problem solving, and collaborative action among formal authorities, citizens at-large, and local opinion leaders around a pressing public matter" (Schoch-Spana et al., 2007). Such community engagement involves two-way communication between governmental officials and community stakeholders who work together to understand each others' perspectives while also tackling complex issues at hand. The end result is a community-based participatory process that considers the potential crisis standards of care that may need to be implemented, with all parties understanding why such standards are necessary and how these standards will be applied within a community context (Schoch-Spana et al., 2007; Bernier, 2009).

Community stakeholders can be divided into (1) healthcare professionals and institutions who would be asked to implement crisis standards of care, and (2) non-healthcare professionals and entities such as patients, family members, or other community laypersons who would be directly impacted by the implementation of such standards of care. Both groups are part of the same community, but specific engagement efforts aimed at both types of community stakeholders, across all phases of disaster planning and response, are necessary to ensure effective engagement and engender trust in the processes and systems put in place (Table 2). Engagement and communication with stakeholders even after a disaster has occurred (the so-called "recovery" phase) is equally important to help stakeholders understand the standards-of- care processes that were employed during the time of crisis as well as to help deal with the aftermath of the crisis scenario.

**TABLE 2** Community and Provider Engagement, Education, and Communication

| Preincident (preparedness) | o | Cultural competency training and linguistically appropriate communications |
| | o | Transparency, engagement, outreach and trust establishment with community-based organizations, faith-based organizations, and community representatives |
| | o | Input into core values or principles to guide standards and implementation |
| | o | Understanding of the fundamental ethical dilemmas involved in decisions that might be made necessary by crisis situations |
| | o | Input on how to avoid the need to implement crisis standards of care, such as through improved understanding and support for a culture of preparedness. |

| Incident (response) | o Establish and promote ongoing communication and situational awareness |
| | o Mental health, palliative care, and bereavement interventions/ provider self-care training |
| | o Develop and communicate resilience strategies |
| | o Ensure equitable care of vulnerable populations |
| Postincident (recovery) | o Mental health screening and interventions |
| | o Continued community engagement and establishment of predisaster clinical roles and patient relationships |
| | o Continued development and promotion of resilience strategies |
| | o Debriefing and learning to facilitate improved future response, including revisions to crisis standards of care as appropriate |

## Preincident Community Engagement

The transition from an individual-based focus to a population-based focus requires federal, state, local, and tribal community level involvement, collaboration, coordination, and cooperation. These governmental entities should reach out to both traditional and non-traditional partners, including new partners in preparedness and response, such as law enforcement, emergency management, and other responders necessary in comprehensive emergency planning and response efforts (Lurie et al., 2006). In partnership, these entities should then work with healthcare providers and their institutions to communicate with and engage community stakeholders in the disaster-planning phase, explaining that crisis standards of care will be applied in disasters during unresolvable circumstances of resource scarcity. While it is important to establish discussions specific to the emergency response topics being considered, it is equally important to work with existing community networks that may already have processes in place that can allow for improved dialogue. Such networks can be made up of a variety of community-based and faith-based organizations, with identification of community leaders to help facilitate the process (ASTHO, 2009). Although community stakeholder engagement can be accomplished through a variety of means in advance of the disaster, the foundation of any such engagement rests on establishing trust among stakeholders anticipated to be involved, including governmental entities, healthcare providers and their institutions, and the lay public. The establishment of trust includes open and honest communication regarding the realities of current resource limitations, scarce resource environments and the impact of catastrophic events on the healthcare system, and its ability to provide the usual level of care that community members otherwise expect. The reasoning behind the decision to implement crisis standards of care in emergency situations must be explained with a high degree of transparency to all stakeholders involved.

This engagement dialogue should be inclusive of the opportunity for community stakeholders to articulate underlying community values and ethical principles of fairness and social justice to ensure that healthcare providers apply these principles appropriately during times of crisis (Houston/Harris County Committee, 2007; Powell et al., 2008; Li-Vollmer, 2009). An example of such an engagement of the public in the preparedness process is the Illinois Faith-Based Pandemic Flu Preparedness ambassador's training program. This program has trained more than 500 faith-based leaders and their congregations in flu preparedness issues, National Incident Management System concepts, and American Red Cross cardiopulmonary resuscitation instruction. This form of engagement is engendering trust, cooperation, and a feeling of partnership among the various stakeholders in the process, setting the stage for further preparedness topics of discussion, such as crisis standards of healthcare delivery. Other examples of organizations engaging communities are the USA Freedom Corps' branch, the U.S. Citizens Corps established after September 11, 2001, and the Medical Reserve Corps and Community Emergency Response Team programs. They have ongoing contributions being made to community response efforts throughout the states (Citizen Corps, 2009).

Every effort should be made to facilitate stakeholder input into the deliberative process because implementation of crisis standards of care will likely require crossing the boundaries of established community ethical, philosophical, religious, legal, and value-based standards. These standards typically exist to protect an individual patient's health and well-being. Discussions about palliative care, dying, and death should be explicit components of this dialogue so that stakeholders can be assured that the healthcare system will not abandon them when resources are scarce. Additional attention should be paid to the disaster mental health needs of both healthcare providers and community stakeholders, with particular focus on those psychological needs that will be accentuated during and after times of crisis.

Governmental leaders and authorities who actively seek community stakeholders and work to understand their perspectives in advance of a disaster are believed to be better able to work with these stakeholders in the midst of a response effort (Schoch-Spana et al., 2007). Thus, while communication and engagement form key components of predisaster planning, it is equally the cornerstone for maintaining understanding and trust during the crisis itself as resource scarcity becomes a stark reality. Building on the trust and credibility that were established during the predisaster phase, governmental entities in partnership with healthcare professionals and institutions will need to provide clear, timely, effective, and appropriate crisis risk communication so that community stakeholders will receive needed ongoing situational awareness of the disaster's impact on precious health system resources as the situation unfolds. Although a number of crisis risk communication tools are available, evaluation of such tools is beyond the scope of this committee's work. However, it should be noted that the CDC's Crisis & Emergency Risk Communication curriculum includes the components of such a strategy and is available for use via the CDC website (CDC, 2009e). Crisis risk communication will assist community stakeholders in understanding their own health risk and help mitigate potential demand on limited system resources, and also help reinforce the predisaster discussions with community stakeholders so they can prepare for the scarce resource situation at hand.

A well-integrated communications plan that is part of an overall disaster response strategy will increase situational awareness, mitigate and address rumors, and ensure that community concerns and anxieties are addressed promptly as the situation unfolds through bidirectional communications (Sheppard et al., 2006; Andrulis et al., 2007). This involves the development of educational materials, emergency messaging, and other systematic strategies by which to disseminate important information to stakeholders including members of the media. Additionally, information about palliative care options and end-of-life care needs should be made an explicit part of the crisis risk communication efforts (Gavagan et al., 2006). Mental health considerations must also play a central role in this communication effort so that individuals (and the community as a whole) can learn to cope with complex disaster mental health concerns tied to crisis standards of care, namely fears, anxiety, perceived or real loss of control, traumatic grief/depression, posttraumatic stress disorder (PTSD), and other disaster-related mental health needs and social changes created by necessary crisis standards of care.

Finally, in addition to improved planning and greater trust, pre-incident community engagement in planning can help create or build alliances and collaborative efforts that aim to avoid the necessity of implementing crisis standards of care. Community engagement can lead to greater support (financial and otherwise) for preparedness efforts, for example.

## Community Engagement to Improve Resiliency

As there are likely to be substantive population-level mental health risks from a mass casualty public health emergency that requires crisis standards of care, there is also an opportunity to promote resilience at the individual and population levels to mitigate these risks. For example, varied crisis standards of care (e.g., allocation of scarce resources, community mitigation strategies) may either be enhanced or bitterly opposed based on levels of public engagement and trust in recommended public health crisis standards of care. Although scant empirical data are available, it is conceivable that desired public behaviors can be enhanced by early and sustained community engagement (Germann et al., 2006; DHHS, 2003). Undesirable (e.g., anti-social or even violent) behaviors and potential social disorganization can be lessened through these efforts, resulting in improved resilience for the individual and the system. Proactive engagement and communications with the public represent a critical opportunity to facilitate individual and community resilience that will hopefully encourage concrete actions they can take now to lessen the potential impacts from events requiring crisis standards of care as well as an ongoing commitment to integrate these issues during response and recovery phases as information changes.

Customized, event-specific risk communications, emergency public health information linked with resilience enhancing psychoeducational coping information, and coping strategies that use social networks to cope with fears and loss may serve to "inoculate" the population and the healthcare workforce from the effects of a mass casualty event requiring crisis standards of care. For example, in a pandemic incident, a key resilience component could be a "Coping with scarce resources/mass casualty events" module disseminated through emergency public information and messaging. Although these population-level behavioral resilience and coping strategies are not currently available, they could be developed to enhance resilience by supporting natural social support systems and expected reactions by facilitating and encouraging natural coping through the use of individual and family "resilience plans"(Schreiber, 2005). In these scenarios, creating mechanisms for supporting and conducting bidirectional communications between the citizenry and public health officials can enhance population-level behavioral resilience. The extent of an enhanced population resilience may have a direct bearing on reducing the surge demand on the healthcare system and other key critical infrastructures on the part of the public and facilitate the willingness of the healthcare workforce to operate under crisis standards of care. Thus, it is important to develop a national platform to support resilience that can customized by communities at the local level.

## Improving Trust with Vulnerable Populations

Building trust is particularly important in more vulnerable populations, including those with preexisting health inequities and those with unique needs related to race, ethnicity, culture, immigration, limited English proficiency, and lower socioeconomic status. Individuals from these communities may have accentuated mistrust for governmental decision making and the healthcare system, and these concerns may parlay into their questioning the fairness and equity of the process during the implementation of crisis standards of care. Concerns for other vulnerable populations such as children, older adults, persons with disabilities, and individuals with medical special needs must also be considered during disaster planning and response because these factors may also impact morbidity and mortality. The needs, challenges, and barriers to caring for these specific community stakeholders must also be considered for integration into the overall disaster response effort *prior* to the implementation of crisis standards of care. Healthcare providers and their institutions should incorporate appropriate cultural competencies to address issues inherent within these disadvantaged communities (Pastor et al., July 2006; Schoch-Spana et al., 2007; Andrulis et al., 2007). A recent collaboration of governmental and non-governmental entities called attention to issues related to working with these populations in an effort to ensure their integration into emergency preparedness and response activities. This culminated in the release of the following National Consensus Statement:

The integration of racially and ethnically diverse communities into public health emergency preparedness is essential to a comprehensive, coordinated federal, state, tribal, territorial, and local strategy to protect the health and safety of all persons in the United States. Such a strategy must recognize and emphasize the importance of distinctive individual and community characteristics such as culture, language, literacy, and trust, and promote the active involvement and engagement of diverse communities to influence understanding of, participation in, and adherence to public health emergency preparedness actions (Drexel University Center for Health Equality, 2008).

Once the crisis has passed, attention should be given to ongoing engagement with community stakeholders to help optimize restoration of function and well-being at both the individual and community levels in the post-recovery phase. Particular attention should be given to mental health triage and needs, especially bereavement, as individuals begin the process of recovery from the dual impacts of both the crisis medical care environment and other non-medical impacts of the incident. Health education, risk communication, community outreach, and other well-established strategies should be incorporated in the recovery phase to ensure that the needs of the community—particularly those from populations that may have been disproportionately impacted during the crisis—are attended to as the medical system returns back toward normalcy (Schoch-Spana et al., 2007).

The community should also be involved in post-incident learning and improvement processes. Trust in the health care system will remain important long after the crisis has passed. Ongoing community engagement offers the opportunity to build and enhance trust, even if incident response did not meet all stakeholders' expectations. Community engagement in the learning process can also offer the benefit of varied insights into the response process and how to improve it.

**Recommendation 3: <u>Seek Community and Provider Engagement</u>**
**State, local, and tribal governments should partner with and work to ensure strong public engagement of community and provider stakeholders, with particular attention to the needs of vulnerable populations and those with medical special needs, in:**

- **Developing and refining crisis standards of care protocols and implementation guidance;**
- **Creating and disseminating educational tools and messages to both the public and health professionals;**
- **Developing and implementing crisis communication strategies;**
- **Developing and implementing community resilience strategies; and**
- **Learning from and improving crisis standards of care response situations.**

## LEGAL ISSUES IN EMERGENCIES

Significant legal challenges may arise in establishing and implementing crisis standards of care. Questions of legal empowerment of various actions to protect individual and communal health are pervasive and complicated by interjurisdictional inconsistencies. The law must inform prevailing standards of care and create incentives for actors to maximize individual and communal health, while also respecting both individual and community rights as much as possible.

### Distinguishing Medical and Legal Standards of Care and Scope of Practice

Modern studies and assessments improve our understanding of how healthcare services change during emergencies to ensure optimal health outcomes (AHRQ, 2005b; GAO, 2008; AMA, 2007; Romig, 2009; Christian et al., 2006; Kanter, 2007). Various actors must be able to organize and effectively use limited medical resources consistent with "crisis" standards of care. Yet, the question of which professional standard changes, whether medical or legal, is less certain. Medical and legal standards of care may be conflated and confused, suggesting a change in one standard automatically leads to a change in the other.

Medical and legal standards of care, however, are not synonymous. *Medical standards of care* describe the type and level of medical care required by professional norms, professional requirements, and institutional objectives (AHRQ, 2005b; Hick, Barbera, and Kelen, 2009; Pegalis, 2009). Medical standards of care vary (1) among types of medical facilities such as hospitals, clinics, and alternate care facilities, and (2) based on prevailing circumstances, including during emergencies. Medical standards of care should not be confused with a healthcare practitioner's scope of practice or associated privileges (Hick et al., 2009; Pegalis, 2009; Curie and Crouch, 2008). Scope of practice refers to the extent of a licensed or certified professional's ability to provide health services pursuant to their competence and license, certification, privileges, or other lawful authority to practice (AHRQ, 2005b; Wise, 2008; Lewandowski and Adamle, 2009).

*Legal standards of care* may be defined as the care and skill that a healthcare practitioner must exercise in particular circumstances based on what a reasonable and prudent practitioner would do in similar circumstances (Mastroianni, 2006; Dobbs, 2000; Hood v Phillips, 1977[1]). Legal standards of care are necessarily flexible according to the fact and situation, and subject to differing interpretations nationally (Dobbs, 2000). Further, the legal standards of care may vary from state-to-state. Yet legal standards of care do not always approximate medical standards. For example, courts assessing standards of care may determine that prevailing medical practice is insufficient or unacceptable in exceptional cases (Canterbury v Spence,1972[2]). Flexibility of the legal standard of care may be beneficial in emergencies, but does not always lend to predictable outcomes when legal disputes arise. This emphasizes the importance of a formal recognition by the state of situations when crisis standards of care are necessary, along with the provision of guidance appropriate to the resource scarcity at issue. Facing uncertainty as to how courts will assess crisis standards of care, healthcare practitioners may react negatively to actual or perceived risks of liability. As discussed below, legal protections may assure healthcare practitioners who act in

---

[1]*Hood v Phillips*, 554 S.W.2d 160 (Tex. 1977).
[2]*Canterbury v. Spence*, 464 F.2d 772 (D.C. Cir. 1972).

good faith that they may not be held liable for their civil wrongs that cause unintended harms to patients during emergencies.

## The Changing Legal Environment During Declared Emergencies

In non-emergencies, existing laws and policies offer reasonable guidance on the empowerment of actors and entities to allocate health resources and deliver health care. During declared states of emergency, however, the legal environment changes (Hodge and Anderson, 2008). Emergency declarations trigger an array of non-traditional powers that are designed to facilitate response efforts through public and private sectors. Emergency laws may (1) provide government with sufficient flexibility to respond; (2) mobilize central commands and infrastructures; (3) encourage response efforts by limiting liability; (4) authorize interstate recognition of healthcare licenses and certifications; (5) allocate healthcare personnel and resources; and (6) help to change medical standards of care and scope of practice (Hodge et al., 2009b).

The extent of legal powers during emergencies, however, depends on the type of emergency declared. The federal government, every state, many territories, and some local governments may declare either general states of "emergency" or "disaster" in response to crises that affect the public's health. Such declarations largely authorize emergency management agencies and others to use general legal powers to coordinate emergency responses. HHS and more than half the states may also declare states of "public health emergency" based in part on the Model State Emergency Health Powers Act (Hodge, 2006; Centers for Law and the Public's Health, 2001). The federal government and some states may declare both states of "emergency or disaster" and "public health emergency," which can lead to confusion as divergent governmental powers and entities seek to respond in overlapping ways.

From these varying emergency declarations arise a host of powers and protections that may impact the setting of standards of care depending, in part, on real-time legal interpretations. Through what has been labeled *"legal triage,"* hospital administrators, emergency planners, EMS providers, public health practitioners, and their legal counsel must prioritize legal issues and solutions to facilitate legitimate public health responses during declared states of emergencies (Hodge and Anderson, 2008). Practicing legal triage is not easy as needs and objectives among agencies during declared emergencies may conflict. Ultimately, however, legal decision making in real-time during emergencies may affect implementation of crisis standards of care.

> **Recommendation 4: <u>Provide Necessary Legal Protec-</u>**
> **<u>tions for Healthcare Practitioners and Institutions</u>**
> **<u>Implementing Crisis Standards of Care</u>**
> **In disaster situations, tribal or state governments should authorize appropriate agencies to institute crisis standards of care in affected areas, adjust scopes of practice for licensed or certified healthcare practitioners, and alter licensure and credentialing practices as needed in declared emergencies to create incentives to provide care needed for the health of individuals and the public.**

*Legal Challenges Concerning Standards of Care in Declared Emergencies*

Healthcare providers responding to public health emergencies involving scarce resources may confront numerous legal challenges, as summarized below. Providers should consult their state and local legal partners (e.g., state Attorney General's office, local government counsel, hospital attorneys) before and during emergencies for additional, specific information due to variations in law and healthcare practice across states.

*Legal Authorization to Allocate Personnel, Resources, and Supplies*

Legal authorization is generally required to shift the provision of care and allocate resources (e.g., personnel, medical supplies, and physical space) during emergencies. Emergency declarations and ensuing orders, as noted above, can be the first step in authorizing such changes and providing liability protections (Louisiana Senate Bill, 2008[3]). Many states' statutory emergency laws, for example, facilitate the recognition of out-of-state healthcare licenses and certificates for the limited duration of a declared emergency to allow for the interstate sharing of healthcare

---

[3]Louisiana Senate Bill No. 301; Act No. 538, §735.3, (2008).

personnel. Memoranda of understanding (MOU) and mutual aid agreements can also facilitate the sharing of health care and other necessary resources when they are scarce during emergencies (Stier, 2009). The Emergency Management Assistance Compact (EMAC) formalizes interstate mutual aid among all 50 states and the District of Columbia (Emergency Management Assistance Compact, 1996[4]). To meet regional and substate resource-sharing concerns, regional, state, county, city, and even local hospital MOUs have also been developed (Hodge et al., 2009a; State of Connecticut, 2006; County of Santa Clara, March 2007; North Central Texas Trauma Regional Advisory Council, 2009).

*Liability Risks and Protections for Healthcare Practitioners*

Liability is a prevalent concern among healthcare providers and entities. This concern may be heightened when providing services during emergencies in which routine healthcare practices and responsibilities change. Potential liability claims against practitioners and entities can result from alleged civil, criminal, and Constitutional violations implicating healthcare providers, volunteers, and government or private entities. Liability may arise from claims of medical malpractice, discrimination, invasions of privacy, or violations of other state and federal statutes (e.g., Emergency Medical Treatment and Labor Act, or EMTALA) (Courtney, 2008). Legal causes of action in disaster are rare, but many healthcare providers and entities remain concerned about their potential exposure to liability risks.

Existing liability protections are often described as a "patchwork" (Swendiman and Jones, 2009; CDC, 2009b). There are no comprehensive national liability protections for healthcare providers or entities in all settings. However, an array of state and federal liability protections exist for providers—particularly volunteers and government entities and officials acting in their official duties—who act in good faith and without willful misconduct, gross negligence, or recklessness (Hoffman et al., 2009; Rosenbaum et al., 2008; TFAH, 2008). Some liability protections, including "Good Samaritan" statutes, Volunteer Protection Acts, and Tort Claims Acts, may apply without an emergency declaration (Centers for Law and the Public's Health, 2004; Hodge, 2006; Volunteer Protec-

---

[4]*Emergency Management Assistance Compact*, Public law 104-321, 104th Congress, 2nd sess. (October, 1996).

tion Act of 1997[5]). Other protections (e.g., those pursuant to EMAC) are triggered by an emergency declaration (Centers for Law and the Public's Health, 2004). Specific declarations, such as those pursuant to the federal Public Readiness and Emergency Preparedness Act, may also provide liability protections (Binzer, 2008). Individuals may also receive special protections when deployed through formalized response teams. More limited liability protections exist for entities and paid, private-sector healthcare workers, although some states also provide immunity for compensated workers (Hoffman et al., 2009; Virginia, 2008[6]; Louisiana Senate Bill, 2008[7]). Additionally, liability protections may stem from the waiver of sanctions for failing to comply with certain federal statutes during emergencies.

This existing patchwork of liability protections can complicate planning and response efforts and deter emergency response participation. Emergency liability protections often have limitations. They might only provide coverage after an emergency declaration and for responders who follow disaster plans or act under government authority, uncompensated volunteers, good-faith acts or omissions, and specified time periods or personnel. In addition, most liability protections do not provide immunity or indemnify practitioners for acts that constitute gross negligence, willful or wanton misconduct, or crimes.

> **Absent national comprehensive liability protections, state and local governments should explicitly tie existing liability protections (e.g., through immunity or indemnification) for healthcare practitioners and entities to crisis standards of care.**

An additional concern of many healthcare practitioners is the extent to which medical malpractice and other forms of insurance will cover medical mistakes or care given outside a provider's scope of practice under crisis standards of care situations. Medical malpractice insurance coverage in declared emergencies differs across states and is dependent on specific insurance policy language. To protect healthcare practitioners from rate increases following frivolous malpractice claims, state law could restrict medical malpractice carriers from increasing premiums of

---

[5] *Volunteer Protection Act*, Public Law 105-19, 42 U.S.C. §14501 *et seq* (1997).
[6] Virginia General Assembly Chapter 507, § 8.01-225.01 (March 16, 2003).
[7] Louisiana Senate Bill No. 301, Act No. 538, §735.3, (2008).

healthcare practitioners who face unsuccessful claims arising from their provision of care in declared emergencies.

> **In considering potential claims of medical malprac-
> tice against healthcare practitioners arising from the
> delivery of health care in declared emergencies,
> courts may (1) take notice of the legal effect of chang-
> ing standards of care during emergencies, and (2)
> consider whether adherence to guidance in this Re-
> port provides sufficient evidence of meeting the stan-
> dard of care.**

*Balancing Individual Legal Rights and Responsibilities and Communal Objectives*

At the core of emergency legal issues is the need to balance individual and communal interests to protect the public's health. Though simply stated, balancing respective legal interests in emergencies is complex (Gostin, 2008). The interests of individuals and the community may conflict, leading to difficult issues in the setting and implementation of crisis standards of care. Due process and other constitutional protections may differ among autonomous adults and children or other wards of the state (e.g., prisoners, persons lacking mental competence) (Gostin, 2008). Non-autonomous individuals may enjoy special Constitutional protections intended to prevent individual harms. For example, government may be legally required to protect the health of minors even though adults may not be similarly protected (Hodge, 2009). At a minimum, all persons enjoy some level of procedural due process related to governmental decisions to establish standards of care. How much process is due under specific circumstances? The key is to balance the public's need to allocate resources in real-time with an individual's right to access available care and assess key decisions. Individual privacy must also be assessed against the need for government or others to provide adequate care or review identifiable health data in health emergencies (Hodge et al., 2004). Decisions concerning standards of care that disproportionately affect individuals on grounds of ethnicity, religion, race, or other protected classes may raise claims of equal protection violations (Gostin, 2008; Swendiman and Jones, 2009).

*Antidiscrimination Protections for Patients*

Discrimination in the provision of health services can also present liability issues during health emergencies. Federal law prohibits discrimination against individuals on the basis of race, color, or national origin (Title VI of the Civil Rights Act of 1964); age (Age Discrimination Act); or disability (Section 504 of the Rehabilitation Act; Americans with Disabilities Act) (Age Discrimination Act of 1975[8]; Americans with Disabilities Act[9]). Violation of these require "rational" documentation as to why this constituted a burden that could not be accommodated. Other forms of discrimination are also prohibited under federal law. Some federal prohibitions may extend to state and local government entities. States may also have their own antidiscrimination laws. Some liability protections will not apply—even during emergencies—to acts of discrimination. Specific limitations on liability or indemnity protections focused on willful or wanton misconduct should be interpreted to include unlawful acts of discrimination.

## OPERATIONAL IMPLEMENTATION OF CRISIS STANDARDS OF CARE

### Clinical Care in Disasters

Disaster events will be marked by a sudden or gradual increase in demand for healthcare services and a related decrease in the supply of resources available to provide such care. This will result in a healthcare-sector response that requires implementation of a variety of "surge capacity" strategies that include steps taken to reduce demand for care (e.g., the implementation of community-based triage capabilities and risk communication about when to seek care) and the augmentation of ambulatory care capacity in addition to better described inpatient care strategies (Hick et al., 2004; Kaji et al., 2006; Barbisch and Koenig, 2006; Davis et al., 2005; Kelen et al., 2006, 2009; California Department of Public Health, 2008 ; Hanfling, 2006). Therefore, all healthcare entities—not just hospitals—should have plans to provide crisis care. Outpa-

[8]*The Age Discrimination Act of 1975*, 42 U.S.C. §§6101-6107 (1975).
[9]*The Americans with Disabilities Act: Allocation of Scarce Medical Resources During a Pandemic*, Title 42 U.S.C. §§ 504 (April 21, 2006).

tient facilities (and community-based clinics, nursing homes, primary care, etc.) may use strategies modified from hospital guidance. EMS agencies may elect to use sample strategies as outlined below or develop system-specific responses.

A number of strategies can be used to bolster the supply of key resources (i.e., space to deliver care, clinical staffing availability, and the availability of key supplies) (Hick et al., 2009; Kaji et al., 2006; Hick et al., 2009). Most likely the crisis will occur over a spectrum of supply and demand spikes, suggesting that a continuum of care will be in place over the course of any disaster response. It may be helpful to consider that surge capacity following a mass casualty incident falls into three basic categories, depending on the magnitude of the event: conventional, contingency, and crisis surge capacity (Box 2). Note that the same event may result in conventional care at a major trauma center, but crisis care at a smaller, rural facility.

Conventional, contingency, and crisis care represent a continuum of patient care delivered during a disaster event. As the imbalance increases between resource availability and demand, health care—emblematic of the healthcare system as a whole— maximizes conventional capacity, then moves into contingency, and, once maximized, moves finally into

---

**BOX 2**
**Conventional, Contingency, and Crisis Capacity**

**Conventional capacity**–The spaces, staff, and supplies used are consistent with daily practices within the institution. These spaces and practices are used during a major mass casualty incident that triggers activation of the facility emergency operations plan.

**Contingency capacity**–The spaces, staff, and supplies used are not consistent with daily practices, but provide care that is *functionally equivalent* to usual patient care practices. These spaces or practices may be used temporarily during a major mass casualty incident or on a more sustained basis during a disaster (when the demands of the incident exceed community resources).

**Crisis capacity**–Adaptive spaces, staff, and supplies are not consistent with usual standards of care, but provide sufficiency of care in the setting of a catastrophic disaster (i.e., provide the best possible care to patients given the circumstances and resources available). Crisis capacity activation constitutes a *significant* adjustment to standards of care (Hick et al., 2009).

crisis capacity. Concurrent with this transition along a surge capacity continuum is the realization that the standard of care will shift. This occurs primarily as a result of the growing scarcity of human and material resources needed to treat, transport, and provide patient care. The goal of the healthcare agency or facility is to return as quickly as possible to conventional care by requesting resources or transferring patients out of the area, drawing on the resources of partner or coalition hospitals and the health system as a whole. Along the span from conventional to crisis care, healthcare facilities should attempt to minimize changes that significantly impact patient outcomes by changing work practices in order to focus resources on patient care (Phillips and Knebel, 2007; ANA, 2008; Gebbie et al., 2009) (Figure 1).

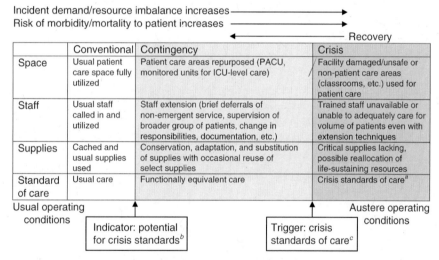

**FIGURE 1** Continuum of incident care and implications for standards of care.
NOTE: Post anesthesia care unit (PACU); intensive care unity (ICU)
[a]Unless temporary, requires state empowerment, clinical guidance, and protection for triage decisions and authorization for alternate care sites/techniques. Once situational awareness achieved, triage decisions should be as systematic and integrated into institutional process, review, and documentation as possible.
[b]Institutions consider impact on the community of resource use (consider "greatest good" versus individual patient needs – e.g., conserve resources when possible), but patient-centered decision making is still the focus.
[c]Institutions (and providers) must make triage decisions balancing the availability of resources to others and the individual patient's needs – shift to community-centered decision-making.
SOURCES: Adapted from Hick et al. (2009); Wynia (2009).

Catastrophic events will have an impact on the entire healthcare delivery "system" and will affect response and delivery of care that occurs in the home, community, hospitals, primary care offices, and long-term care facilities. A number of strategies can be implemented along this continuum of care delivery to reduce the likelihood that standards of care will change in a disaster situation. These include steps taken to substitute, conserve, adapt, and reuse critical resources, including the way staff are used in delivering care. All these steps should be attempted prior to the reallocation of critical resources in short supply (Tables 3 and 4). Every attempt must be made to maintain usual practices and the expected standard of care and patient safety (Rubinson et al., 2008; Minnesota Department of Health, 2008).

**TABLE 3** Sample Strategies to Address Resource Shortages

|  | Conventional Capacity | Contingency Capacity | Crisis Capacity |
|---|---|---|---|
| Prepare | Stockpile supplies used | | |
| Substitute | Equivalent medications used (narcotic substitution) | | |
| Conserve | Oxygen flow rates titrated to minimum required, discontinued for saturations > 95% | Oxygen only for saturations < 90% | Oxygen only for respiratory failure |
| Adapt | | Anesthesia machine for mechanical ventilation | Bag valve manual ventilation |
| Reuse | Reuse cervical collars after surface disinfection | Reuse nasogastric tubes and ventilator circuits after appropriate disinfection | Reuse invasive lines after appropriate sterilization |
| Reallocate | | Reallocate oxygen saturation monitors, cardiac monitors, only to those with critical illness | Reallocate ventilators to those with the best chance of a good outcome |

SOURCE: Adapted from Hick et al. (2009).

**TABLE 4** Sample Strategies for Emergency Medical Services (EMS) Agencies to Address Resource Shortages

| EMS Agency Resources | Contingency Changes | Crisis: Implement Contingency Changes Plus: |
|---|---|---|
| Dispatch | Assign single agency responses, use medical priority dispatch to decline services to select calls | Assign EMS only to life-threatening calls by predetermined criteria, no response to cardiopulmonary resuscitation-in-progress calls, questions may be altered to receive limited critical information from caller |
| Staffing | Adjust shift length and staffing patterns | One medical provider per unit plus driver |
| Response | "Batch" calls (multiple patients transported), closest hospital destination | No resuscitation on cardiac arrest calls, decline service to noncritical, nonvulnerable patients and to critical patients with little to no chance of survival |

Broadening surge capacity must incorporate the full spectrum of patient care delivery capabilities in a disaster-impacted community. This includes planning for extension of hospital-like services in an unregulated, non-healthcare setting. Examples of this include the establishment of Federal Medical Stations (FMSs) during the responses to the multiple Florida hurricanes in summer 2004, Hurricanes Katrina and Rita in 2005, and Hurricanes Gustav and Ike in 2008 (HHS, 2009). The initial concepts for such planning came from work conducted for the U.S. Army Soldier Biological Chemical Command in the late 1990s. These efforts focused on a combination of out-of-hospital capabilities divided between Neighborhood Emergency Help Centers (NEHCs) and Acute Care Centers (ACCs) (Church, 2001a, 2001b; Skidmore et al., May 2003; AHRQ, December 2004; Hamilton et al., 2009a; Hamilton et al., 2009b; Gavagan et al., 2006).

The NEHC is intended to function as a community care station that provides a combination of functions, including victim triage, and serves as a distribution point for medical countermeasures. The ACC, similar to the FMS concept, serves as an out-of-hospital medical treatment facility for patients requiring a lower acuity level of care than that supported in a hospital critical care setting, but not well enough to be managed at home. Pandemic influenza planning has galvanized many communities to adopt such an approach to surge capacity planning, largely based on this theoretical framework (Cinti et al., 2008). The components of this alternate care system are built around a stratification of care model, with emphasis on the use of triage algorithms that prioritize use of community-based services for selective patient care delivery that might otherwise be managed under non-disaster circumstances in the hospital setting. The committee has made the assumption that the delivery of care in an unregulated environment would be construed as an alteration to the existing standard of care. Yet such an approach may be necessary in order to prevent collapse of overburdened hospitals responding to a surge event. Even absent the threat of collapse, in some circumstances (such as an infectious epidemic) it is possible that higher quality, safer care can be provided outside the usual venues for most patients. In such conditions, a decision to relocate most care from hospital emergency departments to alternate care facilities would comprise a change in the usual standard of care, but superior quality compared to attempting to maintain ordinary use of the usual facilities.

## Disaster Mental Health Crisis Standards of Care

In major disaster and emergencies, there will also be a surge of psychological casualties among those directly affected, including responders, healthcare practitioners, and members of the population who have not experienced direct impact. Mass psychological casualties and morbidity will occur in those who experience an aggravation of a prior or concurrent mental health condition. New substantial burdens of clinical disorders, including PTSD, depression, and substance abuse may also arise among those with no prior history. Even in those with no formal disorder, there may be significant distress at a population level, resulting in unparalleled demands on the mental health system.

The magnitude of new incidence disorder in the population has typically ranged from 30 to 40 percent or more in those directly impacted, such as those who experienced personal losses (IOM, 2003; Galea et al., 2005). Although resilience may also be a result for some, the population-level impact of mass casualty incidents compared to other types of disaster will likely result in an substantive mental health burden on the nation during and after use of crisis standards of care requiring mental health interventions across varied "disaster systems of care" including the healthcare system, public and private mental health systems, schools, and coroner and other key systems at the community level (Schreiber, 2005).

Therefore, it is necessary to use a mass casualty disaster mental health concept of operations to enable a crisis standard of disaster mental health care through the use of currently available evidence-based mental health rapid triage and incident management systems. For example, such systems used by the American Red Cross and Los Angeles (LA) County Emergency Medical Services Agency and those recommended by the National Biodefense Science Board Disaster Mental Health workgroup may serve as models (HHS, November 2008). The latter system, known as "PsySTART," provides for rational allocation and alignment of limited acute- and response-phase mental health assets to those with greatest evidence-based risks and needs in a phased, sequential manner so that those in need are matched to resources in the most timely fashion during response and recovery (Thienkrua et al., 2006). In the Los Angeles County Emergency Medical Services agency pilot project, for example, Los Angeles's network of 14 Disaster Resource Center Hospitals (Level 1 trauma centers), the Department of Mental Health, and other key "disaster systems of care" collect and are able to share triage information for near real-time situational awareness and a "common operating picture." This information guides prioritization of crisis intervention at the hospitals and facilitates mutual aid across NIMS levels. Those with the greatest triaged needs are matched to available care until all those who are at risk and desire services can be further assessed and linked in the most timely manner to definitive care (Schreiber, 2005). There is now evidence that certain types of psychological interventions are the treatments of choice for conditions such as PTSD that are a frequent result from disasters, and the triage system allows for faster matching of the high-risk subset to appropriate and timely care (IOM, 2007).

## Palliative Care Planning for Crisis Standards of Care

The provision of palliative care in the context of a disaster with scarce resources is a relatively new component of disaster planning. The goal of palliative care is to prevent and ease suffering and to offer patients and their families the best possible quality of life at any stage of a serious or life-threatening illness and is not dependent on prognosis. It can also be provided at the same time as curative and life-prolonging treatment.

Although the primary goal of a coordinated response to a disaster incident should be to maximize the numbers of lives saved, a practical plan also must provide the greatest comfort for those who will live for awhile before dying as a result of the incident (Holt, 2008). Triage and treatment practices that focus on maximizing the number of lives saved means that during a crisis, some people who might be successfully treated or cured under normal circumstances will die. During a crisis, palliative care would provide aggressive treatment of symptoms, such as pain and shortness of breath. In addition, triage to palliative care should allow for the fact that the initial prognosis for some patients will change, whether by virtue of their doing better than expected or by additional treatment resources becoming available.

Identifying transition points in the condition of patients helps the patient, family, and healthcare providers prepare for the final stage of life. A transition point can be defined as an event in the trajectory of an illness that moves the patient closer to death. For example, a patient with chronic obstructive pulmonary disease may have no change in her condition until she gets influenza and never fully recovers; for that patient, contracting influenza is a transition point in her condition (Berry and Matzo, 2004). Prognostication, aided by a risk index or scale, enables healthcare practitioners to plan clinical strategies during a crisis situation. These tools may be helpful in determining whether a patient's illness has reached a terminal phase (Box 3) (Matzo, 2004).

Providing a treatment category of "palliative care" for those not likely to survive will be an important service option for responders and triage officers. Acknowledging that a patient is not likely to survive typically leads to discussions regarding the goals of care, appropriateness of interventions, and efforts to help the patient and family begin to say good-bye (Matzo, 2004).

When resources are scarce, planners can make available alternative means of palliative care delivery and treatment. Planners should:

- Develop evacuation plans for existing and new palliative care patients;
- Develop a community response plan, staffing plans, and training programs for first responders and other relevant medical personnel;

- Establish transparent, community-based, and explicit triage criteria for casualties not likely to survive;
- Develop a community education program to prepare the public;
- Stockpile needed palliative care medications and supplies (Wilkinson and Matzo, 2006); and
- Participate in disaster planning, response and recovery training, and public education (Holt, 2008).

---

**BOX 3**
**Palliative Care Triage Tools**

**Flacker Mortality Score:** Flacker and Kiely developed a model for identifying factors associated with one-year mortality (the probability of death within the next year) by conducting a retrospective cohort study using Minimum Data Set (MDS) information from residents in a 725-bed, long-term care facility (Flacker and Kiely, 1998). The Flacker Mortality Score instrument is the risk-assessment scale developed from those findings. It is used in conjunction with MDS data collected using the standard Resident Assessment Instrument and is applicable to *elders living in long-term care facilities* (Matzo, 2004; CMS, 2002).

**Risk Index for Older Adults:** The Risk Index for Older Adults establishes point scores for several risk factors associated with death within one year of hospital discharge and allows a clinician to evaluate a patient's risk of death accordingly. The point system is based on a study of 2,922 patients discharged from an acute care hospital (Walter et al., 2001). The researchers concluded that, in predicting one-year mortality, this index performed better than other prognostic scales that focus only on coexisting illnesses or physiologic measures. It takes into consideration a cancer diagnosis and is *applicable to hospitalized elders* (Matzo, 2004).

**Mortality Risk Index:** A recent study by Mitchell and colleagues identified factors associated with the 6-month mortality of nursing home residents diagnosed with advanced dementia (Mitchell et al., 2004). The retrospective study of MDS data from 11,430 patients with advanced dementia admitted to nursing homes in New York and Michigan generated risk scores based on 12 MDS variables. The researchers concluded that these risk scores provided more accurate estimates of 6-month mortality than those derived from existing prognostic guidelines (Matzo, 2004).

---

**Crisis Standards of Care Indicators**

Resources that are likely to be scarce in a crisis care environment and may justify specific planning and tracking include:

- Ventilators and components
- Oxygen and oxygen delivery devices
- Vascular access devices
- Intensive care unit (ICU) beds
- Healthcare providers, particularly critical care, burn, and surgical/anesthesia staff (nurses and physicians) and respiratory therapists
- Hospitals (due to infrastructure damage or compromise)
- Specialty medications or intravenous fluids (sedatives/analgesics, specific antibiotics, antivirals, etc.)
- Vasopressors/inotropes
- Medical transportation

Implementation of crisis standards of care first requires recognition of a resource shortfall or impending resource shortfall. However, good situational awareness and incident management can often forestall any requirement to adjust standards of care as patients can either be moved to areas with resources or resources can be brought in to ameliorate the shortage prior to significant consequences for the patient(s). The committee recognizes that this is a particularly important issue for rural healthcare facilities. This is facilitated by monitoring critical resources and evolving events (e.g., ICU bed availability, ventilator availability, and other external health system measures such as situational awareness of both illness and injury numbers and rates within the community, epidemic curve modeling, etc.) for *indicators* of the need for additional resources or, if no resources are available and no adaptive strategies can be implemented, planning for crisis standards of care. If there is a "no-notice" event such as a major explosion, or indicators are not available (or adjustments are not made or not able to be made), *trigger* events may occur (Box 4).

Indicators such as bed availability are tracked routinely by many hospital systems, and surveillance tools monitor other data streams to provide possible early clues to an evolving epidemic. In addition to

```
┌─────────────────────────────────────────────────────────────┐
│                            BOX 4                              │
│                    Indicators and Triggers                    │
│                                                               │
│  Indicator—measurement or predictor that is used to recognize │
│  capacity and capability problems within the healthcare       │
│  system, suggesting that crisis standards of care may become  │
│  necessary and requiring further analysis or system actions   │
│  to prevent overload.                                         │
│                                                               │
│  Trigger—evidence of use of crisis standard-of-care practices │
│  that require an institutional, and often regional, response  │
│  to ameliorate the situation.                                 │
└─────────────────────────────────────────────────────────────┘
```

event-specific data tracking (e.g., ventilators), these indicators should be used where available to determine the "cushion" within the healthcare system and its variability over time.

Facility, local, and regional indicators should be developed to enable anticipation and management of an incident prior to resources being overwhelmed. When event information is not available before it occurs, a system should be in place to collect/share that information during an event. Indicators may also be needed in the out-patient, homecare, and other environments, but have not yet been described.

The committee was unable to identify evidence that specific indicators have predictive value for intervention (Schultz and Koenig, 2006; Davidson et al., 2006; McCarthy et al., 2006), thus, the indicators noted in this document represent expert opinion only, and should be the subject of further research. Due to variables in staffing, in-patient census, and system characteristics, there were no data points that qualified as "triggers" for automatic action absent a sudden overwhelming event that would not require indicators to recognize. The members did feel strongly, however, that waiting for hard "trigger" evidence of crisis care was inappropriate, and that the goal should be anticipation of resource shortages based on situational awareness (including tracking of indicators), with correction of the problem prior to crisis when possible. The numbers reflected in the table are examples only, as there is tremendous variability between regions (Table 5). For example, at the workshop hosted by the committee some panelists believed that one hospital on ambulance diversion should be an indicator, while others noted that multiple hospitals were on diversion on a routine basis in their communities.

**TABLE 5** Possible Indicators for Crisis Capacity[a]

| Indicators | Institution/Agency | Region | State |
|---|---|---|---|
| Situational awareness indicators | | | |
| Overall hospital bed availability | < 5% available or no available beds for >12 hours | < 5% | < 5% |
| Intensive care unit bed availability | None available | < 5% regional beds available | < 5% state beds available |
| Ventilators | < 5% available | < 5% available | < 5% available |
| Divert status | On divert > 12 hours | > 50% EDs on divert | > 50% EDs on divert |
| Emergency medical services call volume | 2 times usual | | |
| Syndromic predictions | Will exceed capacity | Will exceed capacity | Will exceed capacity |
| Emergency department (ED) wait time | > 12 hours | | |
| Event-specific indicators | | | |
| Illness/injury incidence and severity | | | |
| Disaster declaration | | > 1 area hospital | > 2 major hospitals |
| Contingency care being provided and unable to rapidly address shortfall | Any hospital reporting | Any hospital reporting | Any hospital reporting |
| Resource-specific shortage (e.g., antibiotic, immuno globulin, oxygen, vaccine) | Notification by supplier | Notification by hospitals | Notification by hospitals/suppliers |
| Outpatient care | Marked increase in appointment demand or unable to reach clinic due to call volume | | |
| Staff illness rate | > 10% | > 10% | > 10% |
| School absenteeism | Not applicable | > 20% | > 20% |

| Indicators | Institution/Agency | Region | State |
|---|---|---|---|
| Disruption of facility or community infrastructure and function | Utility or system failure | > 1 hospital affected | > 5 hospitals affected or critical access hospital affected |

[a]The indicators in this table should be developed in relation to usual resources in the area and usage patterns—*numbers are examples only.*

There was agreement with the panelist that *18* hospitals on divert during the severe heat wave in Chicago certainly met the qualification of "indicator" (Stein-Spencer, 2009). In addition, staff absenteeism is likely to affect rural facilities and services disproportionately more than larger urban facilities, and "indicator" thresholds for the impact of infrastructure damage also will vary substantially. Despite the lack of specificity available to the committee, we describe opportunities for indicator capture in the hopes that further study may allow better definition of meaningful thresholds that may have at least some applicability across different populations. In particular, the committee acknowledges that triggers to move to crisis standards of care will likely be different for rural versus urban regions of a state. Therefore, this issue needs to be considered when formulating crisis standards of care protocols for use in disaster situations.

Trigger events revolve around changes to staff, space, and supplies that constitute a change in standard practices such that morbidity and mortality risks to the patient increase (i.e., to crisis standards of care). Trigger events do not necessarily require a state response. If the institution rapidly receives victims from a bomb blast that result in temporary (hours) use of cots for stable patients, but is able to return to conventional operations quickly, the facility can manage this incident internally without the need for the declared crisis standards of care. However, most such incidents require engagement of other healthcare facilities to distribute patients to hospitals with more adequate resources. An example is the 2003 Rhode Island nightclub fire, when manual ventilation of patients was performed in hallways pending air evacuation to regional burn centers (Dacey, 2003). Only in the case that the trigger event(s) are unable to be ameliorated by patient evacuation or resource acquisition is state action required to provide protections to providers who are now delivering care under crisis conditions. This may occur in catastrophic events causing significant infrastructure loss and impeding patient transport (major hurricane or earthquake) or an epidemic (e.g., pandemic) that affects all institutions.

Trigger points are only reached when the institutional surge capacity cannot accommodate the demand through conventional or contingency responses that do not require an adjusted standard of care (Table 6). Trigger points and actions taken when they occur can be easily incorporated into job action sheets or surge capacity templates used at a hospital (e.g., "if providing cot-based care, hospital must notify Regional Medical Coordination Center (RMCC) by calling [555-555-5555]"). Regional personnel monitoring indicators and triggers must also have easy, intuitive, scripted responses to a notification. Some regions may use categorical systems, but these require significant training and maintenance to be effective and understood, and are best used in well-developed, metropolitan systems (University of California, Davis, et al., 2009).

**TABLE 6** Possible Triggers for Adjusting Standards of Care

| Category | Trigger |
| --- | --- |
| Space/structure | Non-patient care locations used for patient care (e.g., cot-based care, care in lobby areas) or specific space resources overwhelmed (operating rooms) and delay presents a significant risk of morbidity or mortality; or disrupted or unsafe facility infrastructure (damage, systems failure) |
| Staff | Specialty staff unavailable in timely manner to provide or adequately supervise care (pediatric, burn, surgery, critical care) even after call back procedures have been implemented |
| Supply | Supplies absent or unable to substitute, leading to risk to patient of morbidity (including untreated pain) or mortality (e.g., absence of available ventilators, lack of specific antibiotics) |

## Crisis Standards of Care Implementation Criteria

Prior to implementation of formal resource triage, the following conditions must be met or in process (Devereaux et al., 2008b):

- Identification of critically limited resources and infrastructure
- Surge capacity fully employed within healthcare facility
- Maximal attempts at conservation, reuse, adaptation, and substitution performed
- Regional, state, and federal resource allocation insufficient to meet demand
- Patient transfer or resource importation not possible or will occur too late to consider bridging therapies
- Request for necessary resources made to local and regional health officials
- Declared state of emergency (or in process)

## Crisis Standards of Care Triage

Triage occurs routinely in medicine, when resources are not evenly distributed or temporarily overwhelmed. Examples include transfer of a patient to a trauma or burn center because most hospitals do not specialize in these types of care, or a mass casualty incident when priority must be assigned for diagnostic imaging or surgery. These decisions are generally ad hoc, based on provider expertise, and have minimal effects on patient outcome. Thus standards of care are routinely adjusted to resources available to the provider without requiring a formal process or declarations. However, the situation in disasters is more complex, as services the hospital usually provide may not be available or not available at all due to demand, with severe consequences to the patient who does not receive these resources.

Triage involves both an assessment of the patient's condition and the available resources. Triage of patients may occur at three points over the course of patient care: (1) primary triage—triage of patients at first contact with the medical system (dispatch, EMS, or emergency department, at which point patients are assigned an acuity level based on the severity of their illness/disease); (2) secondary triage—reevaluation of the patient's condition after initial medical care (this may occur at the scene of

## Prerequisite Command, Control, and Coordination Elements

The implementation of crisis standards of care and fair and equitable resource allocation requires attention to the core elements of incident management, including situational awareness, incident command, and adequate communication and coordination infrastructure and policies. Without this foundation, medical care will be inconsistent, and resources will not be optimally used (Hick et al., 2009).

*Situational Awareness*

Situational awareness will improve the ability to predict and recognize resource shortages and allocate fairly to minimize disparities. Each institution in coordination with community and institution partners should be actively engaged in gathering, interpreting, assessing, and sharing information. Healthcare systems can use multiple sources for information gathering and establish working partnerships prior to crisis events that are then used fully during the crisis.

Information sources or areas for which information is gathered include, but are not limited to:

- Media: television, print, radio, and the Internet;
- Environmental sources of information: reports regarding weather, air, and water quality, etc.;
- Federal communications;
- State and local/regional infrastructure: facility environment of care and community infrastructure (power, telecommunications, road systems, schools, etc.);
- Transportation: mass transit, air transport, port authorities, and information about EMS transportation capabilities, including rotor-wing and ground units; and
- Healthcare systems information: syndromic surveillance, epidemiological monitoring of illness and injury, national pharmacy data, 911 dispatch, call centers, poison control centers, HAvBED, local bed reporting systems, mortuary data, veterinary data, emergency department visits/status, and regional hospital operational and diversion status (AHRQ, 2005a).

Consistent, timely, and two-way information sharing is essential. Established points of contact and means of contact should be exercised regularly.

*Incident Management: Consistency, Coordination, and Communications*

Incident management systems in the United States are based on a common framework called the National Incident Management System. The widely used Hospital Incident Response System is a NIMS-compliant incident management system modified for hospital applications (FEMA, 2009a; California Emergency Medical Services Authority, 2007). All healthcare facilities and entities must have a well-practiced incident management system and understand their plans for notification, activation, mobilization of resources, and continuity of operations.

Health and medical response is managed in the National Response Framework as outlined in Emergency Support Function (ESF) #8—Public Health and Medical Services (FEMA, 2009b; Courtney et al., 2009). At this time, ESF-8 does not have specific provisions for crisis standards of care. However, federal response partners should ensure the integration of relevant provisions. A system of a tiered response, ranging from healthcare management asset through federal responses, has been described by HHS and should be used by all hospitals and regional systems and are a core part of catastrophic response planning (Devereaux et al., 2008a; Phillips and Knebel, 2007; Courtney et al., 2009).

All healthcare systems must also understand how their incident management system interacts with that of jurisdictional emergency management and any coalition hospital response partners, including the process for obtaining assistance during an emergency (Figure 2).

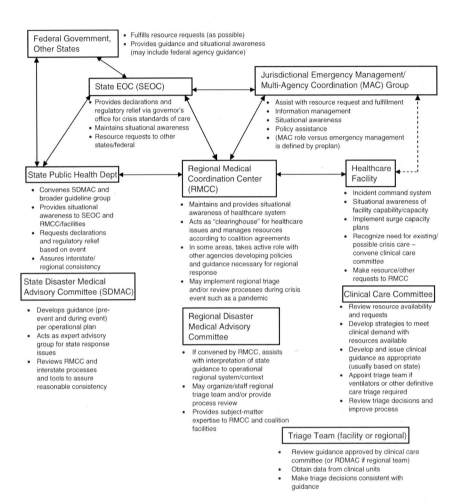

**FIGURE 2** Overview of relationships among agencies, committees, and groups
NOTE: Depending on the organization of the state, the functional layout, details, and relationships among the units might vary.

*Local/Regional Healthcare Coalitions*

In many areas, regional healthcare coalitions exist that provide a common coordination point for hospital planning and response (Courtney et al., 2009; Phillips and Knebel, 2007; Hodge et al., 2009a). In certain environments, this coordination may be supplied by the state. Often, the coalition designates a Regional Medical Coordination Center (RMCC) function that coordinates hospital information and coordinates resource management during a major disaster (Burkle et al., 2007; Courtney et al., 2009; Phillips and Knebel, 2007). These coalitions may be within a jurisdiction, represent an entire jurisdiction, or overlap several jurisdictions or even states. Coalitions are generally organized around functional medical referral areas, however, as noted by Courtney et al. (2009):

> The geographic boundaries of healthcare coalitions are highly variable, and the definition of community must remain flexible to incorporate local needs and realities. The essential feature is that every hospital in the chosen geographic area is included. In some places, the coalition may be composed of all hospitals and other members within a county or a city, while in others members may be from an entire state. In some small or low population density states, a single coalition may represent all hospitals and relevant partners in the entire state. In some large cities, the jurisdiction may be divided into [smaller] more manageable sub-municipal regions, so that a single city might have multiple coalitions. In many locations, coalitions cross jurisdictional borders and are not aligned with the normal geographic boundaries of all individual coalition members.

Healthcare coalitions should be designed to provide added administrative and logistical support to the many components of the health system that need to share limited resources or to transfer patients due to disaster situations. Notably, during a catastrophic disaster, reliance on the state or adjacent regions may become greater. Similar to traffic management or information technology networks, when one part of the system is overloaded, other parts of the system can help accommodate the load and maintain function. During a pandemic, limited or no "buffer" is available due to the pervasive nature of the epidemic, and the coalition function

ian care in an emergency, and are often involved in community-based planning efforts.

*State Coordination*

State coordination often occurs at the state EOC which is the recipient of information provided from the local and regional levels via the local EOC, RMCC(s), and MAC centers. Based on the information provided by the local and regional entities, the state EOC evaluates and processes resource requests. At the state level, resources should be allocated to regions in greatest need during a pervasive event, and guidance provided and emergency power actions taken as needed. This requires excellent ability to gather, coordinate, and communicate information in order to be effective. The state EOC is also the means for relaying information to the local level from neighboring states and the federal partners regarding situational awareness related to resource availability and conditions of medical practice in other regions.

Coordination of care in a disaster event is of paramount importance to the successful mitigation and response effort. This is even more crucial in situations in which there may be a scarcity of resources available for providing care where the overriding state goal is to ensure a level of care across the state that is as consistent as possible. Social chaos and disruption may arise from public perceptions that one community or healthcare system is providing a different level of services than another. This failure to meet public expectations regarding the availability of fundamental healthcare services has the likely effect of exacerbating public confusion during an already chaotic disaster event, while undermining confidence in those responsible for taking charge (Townsend, 2006; Danzig et al., 2007; McHugh et al., 2004).

In addition, one of the fundamental tenets in delivery of healthcare services under crisis conditions is that every effort will be made to maximize delivery of care to a standard that meets community norms, until that is simply not possible. Without the sort of coordination that allows for the visibility of available resources and their location, this cannot occur. Patients cannot be denied resources just because the resources are exhausted in one area, when they are available nearby.

Interstate coordination occurs at the state EOC during an event (via the governor's office or designated agencies such as public health) in order to ensure coordination of resource-sharing agreements, information exchange, and consistent decision implementation related to standards of care. Before the event, such dialogue is the responsibility of the State Department of Health, though local health departments in major metropolitan areas may also need to open dialogue directly with border communities in other states to ensure common assumptions and frameworks.

> **Recommendation 5: <u>Ensure Intrastate and Interstate Consistency Between Neighboring Jurisdictions</u>**
> **States, in partnership with the federal government and localities, should initiate communications and develop processes to ensure intrastate and interstate consistency in the implementation of crisis standards of care. Specific efforts are needed to ensure that Department of Defense, Veterans Health Administration, and Indian Health Services medical facilities are integrated into planning and response efforts.**

## Crisis Standards of Care Operations

When crisis care becomes necessary, a threshold has been crossed requiring that the affected institution(s) either quickly address the situation internally, or, more likely, appeal to partner facilities and agencies for assistance in either transferring patients to facilities with resources or bringing needed resources to the facility. If these strategies cannot be carried out, or if partner facilities are in the same situation (e.g., a pandemic influenza scenario), then systematic implementation of crisis standards of care at the state level may become necessary in order to codify and provide guidance for triage of life-sustaining interventions as well as to authorize care provided in non-traditional locations (alternate care facilities).

Because disaster incidents may have a wide-ranging impact on service delivery, a number of processes must occur, as described below.

### State Responsibilities

The state has an obligation to ensure consistency of medical care to the highest degree possible when crisis care is being provided. Usual coordination and resource requests outlined above are used to minimize healthcare service disruption and/or to provide the most consistent level of care across the affected area and the state as a whole. When prolonged or widespread crisis care is necessary, the state should issue a declaration or invoke emergency powers empowering and protecting providers and agencies to take necessary actions to provide medical care *and* should accompany these declarations with clinical guidance, developed by the State Disaster Medical Advisory Committee (SDMAC), to provide a consistent basis for life-sustaining resource allocation decisions. Individual hospitals and healthcare facilities should work through tactical mutual aid agreements with other local facilities and at the regional level to ameliorate conditions that might force crisis standards of care. When these strategies have been exhausted, healthcare facilities, working through local public health authorities, should request a State emergency declaration recognizing that crisis conditions are at hand, that a change in acceptable standards of care are required, and that crisis standards of care must be initiated.

The SDMAC should be part of the planning process, as outlined in the section above on state planning, but also can be an important part of the response process, drawing on its expertise and that of other pre-identified subject-matter experts to address response-generated issues.

Thus, the state, through its emergency powers, resource allocation, and provision of clinical guidance, attempts to "level the playing field" at the state level, as well as provide legal protections for providers making difficult triage decisions and provide relief from usual regulations that might impede coping strategies such as alternate care facilities.

Regional healthcare coalition data on the status of patient care delivery and access to key resources should be reflected to the state level, where the state EOC synthesizes information. The state EOC will be an important broker of information gathered from across the state, as well as the initial source of relayed information made available from neighboring states and the federal government.

### Regional Responsibilities

Some hospital coalitions cover large metropolitan areas and thus, the Regional Medical Coordination Center acts as liaison between the state and its constituents. The RMCC may be an agency, such as public health, or a hospital or other facility designated by the system. The RMCC attempts to ensure regional medical care consistency and may do so by acting as a resource "clearinghouse" between the healthcare facilities and emergency management and coordinating policy and information to meet regional needs. This may involve a *Regional* Disaster Medical Advisory Committee (RDMAC) or at least a medical advisor or coordinator with access to technical experts in the area, particularly in large metropolitan areas because the specific needs of the area may not be well addressed by state guidance. However, the regional guidance cannot be *inconsistent* with that of the state.

## Healthcare Facility Responsibilities

Though this section will emphasize emergency and hospital-based care, *all* healthcare facilities should have plans to preserve the acute care and other critical elements of their disaster services through elimination of certain usual services and curtailment of others. Taking an approach that incorporates "engineered failure" will ensure that those services that are absolutely essential will be maintained, at the expense of less pressing needs (Hick et al., 2007; ICDRM, 2009). For example, the delivery of dialysis care to patients with end-stage renal disease may be prioritized over out-patient elective surgery. A sample institutional process is outlined in Box 5 below.

## Clinical Care Committee

The individual healthcare institution surge capacity plan should incorporate the use of a "clinical care committee" that is composed of clinical and administrative leaders who can focus a hospital or hospital system approach to the allocation of scarce, life-saving resources (Phillips and Knebel, 2007; Hick and O'Laughlin, 2006; O'Laughlin and Hick, 2008).

---

**BOX 5**
**Sample Institutional Process**[a]

1. Incident commander recognizes that systematic changes are or will be required to allocate scarce facility resources and that no regional resources are available to offset demand.
2. Incident commander activates clinical care committee (or designated members).

3. Planning chief gathers any guidelines, epidemiologic information, resource information, and regional hospital information.
4. Clinical care committee reviews facility/regional situation and examines:
    a. Alternate care facilities—can additional areas of the building or external sites be used for patient care? (should be planned in advance).
    b. Medical care adaptations—(e.g., use of non-invasive ventilation techniques, changes in medicine administration techniques, use of oral medications and fluids instead of intravenous, etc.).
    c. Changes in staff responsibilities—to allow specialized staff to redistribute workload (e.g., floor nurses provide basic patient care in the intensive care unit while critical care nurses "float" and troubleshoot) and/or incorporate other healthcare providers, lay providers, or family members where practical (Rubinson et al., 2008; Rubinson et al., 2005).
    d. Regional challenges and strategies being used by members of the coalition (with ongoing coordination with the Regional Medical Coordination Center and, if used, the Regional Disaster Medical Advisory Committee).

    Develop strategies based on challenges—the committee describes how resources at the facility (emergency department [ED] resources, beds, operating rooms, ventilators) will be allocated. (What level of severity will receive care? What tool or process will be used to make decisions when there are competing demands for the same resource?)
5. Committee summarizes strategies for next operational period and determines meeting and review cycles for subsequent periods (may involve conference calls or similar to avoid face-to-face meetings during a pandemic).
6. Incident commander approves committee strategies as part of incident action plan. Plan is operationalized. Public Information Officer communicates updates to staff, patients, families, and the public.
7. Current in-patients, patients presenting to the hospital, and their family members are given verbal and printed information (ideally by the triage nurse in the ED, or for in-patients, by their primary nurse or physician) explaining the situation and, if necessary, explaining specific resources subject to triage or "treatment trials" that may have to be ended in order to provide care to others with higher likelihood of benefit. A mechanism for responding to patient/family questions and concerns should also be detailed in the written guidance.
8. Security and behavioral health response plans should be implemented.
9. ED/out-patient screening of patients (and denial of service to patients either too sick or too well to benefit from evaluation/admission) based on guidance disseminated by the clinical care team is implemented.
10. Tertiary triage team (ideally NOT the physicians directly providing the patients care and ideally two critical care physicians of equal "rank" in the institution) considers situations in which there are competing patient demands for a scare resource. The resource should be assigned as follows.
    a. When two patients have essentially equal claim to the resource, a "first-come, first-served" policy should be used.

b. When, according to guidelines or the triage team's clinical experience, the claim to the resource is clearly not equal, the patient with a more favorable prognosis/prediction shall receive the resource.

c. The triage team should ask for and receive whatever patient information in necessary to make a decision, but should NOT consider subjective assessments of the quality of the patient's life or value to society and, in fact, should ideally be blinded to such information when possible.

11. The in-patient unit leader (under HICS, or comparable position) should be appointed to make final bed assignments and changes and communicate triage decisions to the clinical team. This individual should have access to real-time-in-patient and out-patient system status and when needed, patient clinical information.

12. Whenever a decision is made to reallocate a ventilator or similar critical resource, the treating physician and family should be provided with the grounds for the decision (which should be documented for the record at the facility), and a rapid appeals process if there is additional or new information that the family or treating physician(s) feel would affect the decision.

13. Transition care plans should assure the comfort and dignity of those who are no longer receiving full treatment modalities and assure support for the family and care providers.

[a]Adapted from Hick et al. (2007).

A clinical care committee is activated by the facility incident commander when the facility is practicing contingency or crisis care due to factors that are not readily reversible. This committee is responsible for making prioritization decisions about the use of resources at the relevant healthcare institution (e.g., hospital, primary care, EMS agency, and others). Some health systems own many facilities in an area, and may have a central committee, with a liaison at each hospital to prioritize within their system. This committee will also inform the institution's incident commander and planning chief about capabilities, recommendations, and requirements for providing care under such conditions. Members should include institution administrators, attorneys, a nursing supervisor, a respiratory care supervisor, ethicists, a community representative, and representatives from relevant clinical departments, though response configurations may be much smaller and tailored to incident needs by the facility incident commander (Hick and O'Laughlin, 2006). Although the institution's clinical care committee's deliberations will be institution focused, the institutional incident commander or planning chief should have some situational awareness of what is occurring outside the institution—in the rest of the health system (e.g., resource demand, disease burden, etc.).

In addition, the institution's clinical care committee must be able to allocate critically limited life-saving interventions. The VHA refers in its guidance to this group as the "Scarce Resource Allocation" committee. The IOM committee prefers "Clinical Care Committee" due to the broader responsibilities this group may take on, but understands that this group may be called different names and achieve the same function (The Pandemic Influenza Ethics Initiative, 2008, 2009).

The clinical care committee chair, in conjunction with the incident command, must maintain active liaison with the RMCC (and RDMAC, if activated) and as needed with the SDMAC to maintain situational awareness of area resources, challenges, strategies, and guidance.

*Triage team*

In some cases, critical life-sustaining resources such as ventilators may have to be triaged in a proactive, systematic fashion consistent with state guidance. In this case, the clinical care committee should appoint or ensure access to a triage team, which will use decision tools appropriate to the event and resource being triaged to make allocation decisions (Devereaux et al., 2008b; AHRQ, 2005b; Hick et al., 2007; Hick et al., 2004; O'Laughlin and Hick, 2008).

The patient's bedside clinician should *not* be the triage decision maker in order to remain an advocate for the patient. The triage team may be located at the hospital or may be a regional function, depending on the preference of the hospital coalition, and its composition may vary somewhat depending on resources available, but generally should be no less than two experienced clinicians (AHRQ, 2005b; Rubinson, 2008b; Tabery and Mackett, 2008). At a regional level, the triage team can provide advice and also help smaller hospitals, and other appropriate components of the health system, to determine the priorities for rural patient transfers and provide advice regarding current status of critical care at larger facilities. Documentation is placed into the patient's record regarding any decisions made by the triage team, including the situation and specific justifications. The triage team's recommendations are then carried out by a nursing supervisor or other designee of the institution, and are reviewed by the clinical care committee on a daily basis for quality and process assurance.

The triage team's decisions may be reviewed more expediently in two cases:

- Clinical review—if the patient's clinical condition has changed significantly since data were supplied to the team, the patient's provider can request a reassessment prior to discontinuation of treatment that the triage team will consider.
- Process review—if there are concerns raised about an unjust or inappropriate application of the triage process, the clinical care committee chair will review the decision-making process. This review may occur before or after withdrawal of treatment, depending on the complaint and when it is received, and a finding will be issued, including communication to a regional or state ethical workgroup or board, depending on the state's structure (The Pandemic Influenza Ethics Initiative, 2008, 2009; DeBruin et al., January 2009).

## Decision Tools and Resource Use Guidance

Decision tools are used by the triage team as a basis for, or to at least inform, triage decisions. Triage decision tools must be regionally consistent in a disaster event, highlighting the importance of the state as a source of guidance when possible. The healthcare coalition RMCC (or RDMAC, if established) can serve as the coordinator of policy, information, and process improvement. Intrastate consistency should be monitored by the SDMAC. The state department of health or governor should assure that the guidance they approve is consistent across state borders by consultation with adjacent state health departments (and EOCs during an event).

State guidance can also offer additional information about maximizing availability of the scarce resource to minimize impact on patients that may be specific to a resource or broader (Minnesota Department of Health, 2008). Decision tools and guidance should not be construed as to prevent reasonable consideration of other clinical factors that may weight a decision to provide or reallocate a scarce resource, but are issued to provide consistency and as much weight of evidence as possible to the decision-making process. This discussion provides a cross-section of available information that was the best available to the committee at the time of writing.

Although the most examined decision tools revolve around mechanical ventilation, guidance is also available for other core medical care components (medications, oxygen, etc.) and limited guidance is available for specific other resources (see Box 6) (Minnesota Department of Health, August 2008). Little guidance is available for the dispatch, EMS, home care, long-term care, and ambulatory care environments as part of the overall health system within a community. Though much of the core component guidance does apply, agencies and entities should examine potential scarce resources and outline coping strategies using base principles similar to those for hospital environments (Rubinson et al., 2008; ANA, 2008). None of the current systems or guidance was designed for pediatrics or other medical special needs patients, and this gap should be addressed by appropriate specialty expert groups. Finally, the needs of other vulnerable populations should also be kept in mind to ensure fairness in the system that is developed.

---

**BOX 6**
**Select Specific Resource Issues**

Note: synopsis and examples are not comprehensive, but suggest areas for state guidance and expert working group efforts.

Blood products—The American Association of Blood Banks can facilitate blood delivery rapidly to areas affected by disasters. However, in the immediate aftermath of a catastrophe, local shortages may occur. Hospital blood banks and their suppliers should determine triage plans ahead of time, altering indications for transfusion and capping use of products where necessary (Schmidt, 2002; Ontario Ministry of Health and Long-term Care, 2008).

Elective surgery triage—Assessment of surgical schedules during an event may require a cancellation of the procedures that are most likely to require postoperative critical care and may assist in opening/maintaining capacity. Determining which procedures may be safely deferred and for how long is important. Ontario's and Utah's plans both include assessments of elective surgeries (Ontario Ministry of Health and Long-term Care, 2008; The Utah Hospitals and Health Systems Association, January 2009).

Trauma care[a]—Catastrophic disasters may produce overwhelming numbers of trauma patients. Most disasters do not overwhelm surgical services, but contingency (conducting temporizing surgical procedures, performing bedside procedures, limiting interventions to patients with good outcome and single-system trauma) and crisis (providing no interventions in the operating room in favor of controlling hemorrhage in multiple patients and performing chest decompression and other limited life and limb-saving interventions) plans should be understood by the surgical and support staff (Eastridge et al., 2006; Propper et al., 2009).

Radiation[a]—Guidelines for triage of radiation incident victims are widely available, though literature and predictive instruments are scant for victims of combined trauma and radiation injury (Waselenko et al., 2004; Fliedner et al., 2001; REMM, 2009; IAEA, 2009). Guidance for response to an improvised nuclear device detonation with more detailed guidance for health and medical response is to be published in 2010 (DHS, January 2009).

Burn care[a]—Care of multiple burn victims requires exceptional amounts of analgesia, intravenous fluids, and burn dressings. However, these may be inexpensively and easily stockpiled. In mass casualty events, an age/percentage burn table has been published as an adjunct for triage decisions (Saffle et al., 2005). Providing care to many victims with limited staff and burn unit space must be addressed in planning (Posner et al., 2003).

Cancer—During a disaster, continued comfort and care appropriate to the resources available should be ensured. Particular emphasis for palliative care needs should be considered in this population. Ontario has published basic guidance to assist with determining priorities for this special population (Ontario Ministry of Health and Long-term Care, 2008).

Renal replacement—Availability of renal replacement therapy may be extremely limited after a disaster due to competing demands for dialysis from incident-related patients or unsafe water supply. Deferral of usual dialysis schedules and indicators may have to occur, and other measures instituted. Ontario has published basic guidance to assist with determining priorities for this special population (Ontario Ministry of Health and Long-term Care, 2008).

Vaccines—Pandemic and other vaccines may initially be in short supply, and priorities may need to be established. Liability and mass vaccination logistic issues may have to be addressed. Guidance for administration will come from the Centers for Disease Control and Prevention, or CDC (e.g., Advisory Committee on Immunization Practice's recommendations for 2009 H1N1 vaccine priority groups). However, further splitting of priority groups may have to occur at the state and even institutional level depending on supply (CDC, 2009c).

Antiviral medications—By example, some medications in relative shortage may be targeted to those at highest risk, those most likely to benefit, or use reduced to prevent evolution of resistance. Limited treatment of 2009 H1N1 with antiviral medication recommendations from the CDC are an example of this form of triage of resources and must be adopted and circulated by the state and voluntarily implemented by providers (CDC, 2009d).

[a]Regional (may be interstate or intrastate) planning should provide for hospitalization of the most critical patients at appropriate centers, with diffusion of less critical victims to community hospitals and transfers used when possible.

Though the "fair innings" argument to allow ventilator allocation to younger patients is attractive at face value, age is not a medically useful predictor of outcome; use of age as a criterion in and of itself also raises ethical and legal concerns. Until society determines through public engagement that age-based triage (or other non-medical criteria such as functional capacity) is appropriate and defines an appropriate range, the committee recommends avoiding age-based criteria. Furthermore, the committee cautions against the prima facie use of DNR status as a decision tool, as underlying, life-limiting medical conditions should primarily be used as triage criteria rather than the fact that the patient has provided an advance directive.

The committee also notes that, although SOFA is useful to assign retrospective survival prediction, it was not designed as a prospective predictor of survival, and thus, differences in a single point on the SOFA scale are of unknown clinical significance for prediction of outcome. This should be considered, particularly when attempting any modification or extension of the SOFA scale beyond its initial construct that may further compromise its predictive value and when using systems that would assign or discontinue a resource based on a single-point change in the SOFA score.

SOFA has not been validated on a pediatric population. Although the principles of increasing mortality with increasing multi-organ dysfunction do apply, caution must be exercised when using SOFA to make anything but broad comparisons. Currently, predictive scoring systems for pediatrics (e.g. PRISM, P-MODS) are being considered for use in performing pediatric triage for ventilator allocation (Pollack et al., 1988; Graciano et al., 2005). However, at least one of these tools, PRISM, involves the evaluation of additional laboratory variables than those required for SOFA, and therefore might be more difficult to apply under conditions of crisis care. The other tool, P-MODS, evaluates parameters different than those used in SOFA scoring. The committee concludes that urgent recommendations from pediatric disaster groups and research are needed to address this gap. Adopters of decision tools should understand their limitations and scope and communicate issues of uncertainty to the triage team members.

The only process and triage system that is the output of an expert, specialty society working group with broad stakeholder input at this time is that of the American College of Chest Physicians (ACCP) (Devereaux et al., 2008b). The advantage of the ACCP process, though less specific than some systems, is that it considers duration of need and underlying disease in addition to the SOFA score acuity assessment. The basic triage process is outlined in Figure 4 and the exclusion criteria are described in Box 7, with additional supportive materials available in the original article. This process has informed most state guidance and other system guidance, including the VHA and other guidelines (Minnesota Department of Health, August 2008; The Pandemic Influenza Ethics Initiative, 2008, 2009; The Utah Hospitals and Health Systems Association, January 2009; Colorado Department of Public Health and Environment, July 2009).

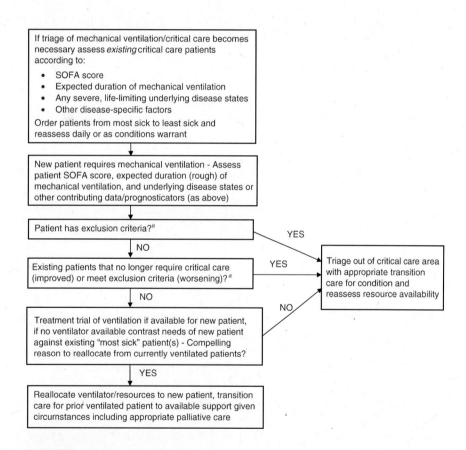

**FIGURE 4** Triage algorithm process.
[a]Example exclusion criteria include severe, irreversible organ failure (CHF, liver, etc), severe neurologic compromise, extremely high or not improving SOFA scores, etc.
SOURCE: Adapted from Devereaux et al. (2008b).

BOX 7
Exclusion Criteria Prompting Possible Reallocation of Life
Saving Interventions

**Sequential Organ Failure Assessment (SOFA) score criteria:** patients excluded from critical care if risk of hospital mortality > 80%
A. SOFA > 15
B. SOFA > 5 for >5 d, and with flat or rising trend
C. > 6 organ failures

**Severe, chronic disease with a short life expectancy**
A. Severe trauma
B. Severe burns on patient with any two of the following:
   i.   Age > 60 yr
   ii.  > 40% of total body surface area affected
   iii. Inhalational injury
C. Cardiac arrest
   i.   Unwitnessed cardiac arrest
   ii.  Witnessed cardiac arrest, not responsive to electrical therapy (defibrillation or pacing)
   iii. Recurrent cardiac arrest
D. Severe baseline cognitive impairment
E. Advanced untreatable neuromuscular disease
F. Metastatic malignant disease
G. Advanced and irreversible neurologic event or condition
H. End-stage organ failure (for details see Devereaux et al., 2008b)
I. Age > 85 yr (see Lieberman et al., 2009)
J. Elective palliative surgery

SOURCE: Adapted from Devereaux et al. (2008b)

> **Critical care and ventilator allocation decision tools should be consistent with currently available evidence-based expert panel and national critical care guidelines, although modifications may be made to meet the specific needs of the state.**

Of note, ventilators may not be the only relevant limitation to mechanical ventilation, as available staff, oxygen, and medication supply may not be able to support significantly more ventilators than the hospital normally uses due to design and supply limitations, thus, wholesale purchase of ventilators may not obviate the issue. Finally, decision tools may be supplemented by event-specific information (e.g., mortality data during a pandemic for particular underlying disease states or age ranges) or by supplemental prognostic information (e.g., as discussed in palliative care section). During an event such as a pandemic, federal guidance may be issued or epidemiologic information may be available that may affect state guidelines.

As evidence improves in triage science, modifications to these recommendations are likely. The state department of health or other appropriate office must maintain an advisory panel that can consider and incorporate necessary updates to this information prior to and during events and provide feedback on or assist with crisis clinical guidance development to ensure that the best available evidence is used should this type of triage be required. These state entities are encouraged to work with localities to ensure that local/regional coordination is occurring in real-time.

**Recommendation 6: <u>Ensure Consistency in Crisis Standards of Care Implementation</u>**
**State departments of health, and other relevant state agencies, in partnership with localities should ensure consistent implementation of crisis standards of care in response to a disaster event. These efforts should include:**

- **Using "clinical care committees," "triage teams," and a state-level "disaster medical advisory committee(s)" that will evaluate evidence-based, peer-reviewed critical care and other decision tools and recommend and implement decision- making algorithms to be used when specific life-sustaining resources become scarce.**
- **Providing palliative care services for all patients, including provision of comfort, compassion, and maintenance of dignity.**
- **Mobilizing mental health resources to help communities—and providers themselves—to manage the effects of crisis standards of care by following a concept of operations developed for disasters;**

- **Developing specific response measures for vulnerable populations and those with special medical needs, including pediatrics, geriatrics, and persons with disabilities.**
- **Implementing robust situational awareness capabilities to allow for real-time information sharing across affected communities and with the "disaster medical advisory committee."**

## CONCLUSION

The potential tragedy wrought by catastrophic disaster, whether naturally occurring or due to intentional acts, should serve as a clarion call to political leadership, policy makers, disaster planners, and the community at large to carefully plan for the allocation of scarce resources efficiently and fairly. Under circumstances in which demand for care exceeds supply, access to a broad continuum of healthcare resources—including those required for life-sustaining intervention—may be curtailed. Disaster events may challenge the depth of human, materiel, and intellectual resources required to respond to them. A highly pathogenic pandemic, detonation of a nuclear weapon, destructive earthquake, or severe hurricane could each pose challenges to the delivery of health care beyond the "imaginable." For this reason, it is imperative that as a nation, we consider our response to such events, ensuring that the processes we use to triage the delivery of care meet the highest ethical standards, and are based on the humanitarian imperative that "all possible steps should be taken to prevent or alleviate human suffering arising out of...calamity, and that civilians so affected have a right to protection and assistance" (The Sphere Project, 2004). In addition, while all populations remain vulnerable to catastrophic events particular populations remain more vulnerable than others. These populations—as described in the committee's report—should be given particular attention to make sure their unique needs are considered in disaster planning and response efforts. As such, the Committee supports the efforts of the World Health Organization and similar agencies in affirming the importance of addressing health inequities and the social determinants of health because those most vulnerable in communities prior to a disaster are those most likely to be impacted adversely by the disaster itself (WHO, 2008).

A number of overarching, guiding principles that were first elucidated in 2004 (AHRQ, 2005b) remain relevant in the discussion of this complex topic and were considered by the committee:

- Allocation of scarce resources is ultimately intended to preserve the functioning of the healthcare system, and to deliver the best care possible under emergency circumstances.
- Planning for the health and medical response to a catastrophic, mass casualty event must take a regional, systems approach, and involve a broad array of public and private community stakeholders.
- Adequate ethical and legal frameworks must be in place that protect both the rights of patients and the rights of those providing care to patients, despite the austere conditions under which such care is being delivered.
- Active engagement of the public is essential; transparent communication of the complexities and challenges related to disaster responses must occur before, during, and after any catastrophic event to mitigate the potential for social disorganization and to promote community resilience.

Crisis standards of care, as described in this report, will be required when the intent and ability to provide usual care is simply no longer possible due to the circumstances. As acknowledged by the committee, some governments have made great strides in determining how to approach resource scarcity, but much work remains to be done.

Indeed, the committee highlighted a number of areas worthy of further discussion, evaluation, and study. Some of these issues constitute real or perceived barriers that will make the implementation and operationalization of crisis standards of care difficult to achieve. Some simply reflect the fact that the study of this area of disaster medicine remains an evolving pursuit requiring multidisciplinary participation. Nonetheless, the discussion around this topic has matured tremendously in the past few years. Despite the gaps that remain (see Table 8), the committee is greatly encouraged by the search for solutions that are taking place.

In studying this issue, the committee's intent is to provide a framework that allows consistency in describing the key components required by any effort focused on standards of care in a disaster. It also intends that, by suggesting such uniformity, consistency will develop across jurisdictions, regions, and states so that this guidance will be useful in con tributing to a uniform national framework for responding to crisis in a fair, equitable, and transparent manner.

**TABLE 8** Impediments to Crisis Standards of Care Implementation

| Key Elements | Gaps to Crisis Standards Implementation |
|---|---|
| Ethical elements | o Articulation of community values and preferences regarding allocation of scarce resources<br>o Consultation and education for practitioners and community about which actions are ethically justifiable during crisis standards, and which are not |
| Community and provider engagement | o Absence of public and stakeholder discussion framework<br>o Absence of "clearinghouse" repository for collected works<br>o Financial impact of resource-sparing strategies<br>o Financial commitments for community engagement/education processes<br>o Incomplete, inconsistent regional partnership development |
| Legal authority and environment | o Inconsistent liability protections<br>o Inconsistent application of scope of practice<br>o Uncertainty about existing liability protections<br>o Uncertain role of community "informed consent" |
| Indicators and triggers | o Limited situational awareness and real-time information exchange |
| Clinical process and operations | o Limited evidence base for select population groups (pediatrics, geriatrics)<br>o Uncertain expectations for completion of diminished documentation<br>o Uncertain process for deescalation from crisis care to conventional care (return to "normalcy")<br>o Uncertain processes for developing constructive after-action reports documenting crisis care responses<br>o Uncertain strategy for using community-based assets of the health system (i.e., private practices, ambulatory care clinics) in managing a crisis surge response<br>o Lack of meaningful/realistic exercise opportunity to evaluate scarce resource planning |

# A

# References

AHRQ (Agency for Healthcare Research and Quality). 2004. *Rocky Mountain regional care model for bioterrorist events: Locate alternate care sites during an emergency.* http://www.ahrq.gov/research/altsites.htm (accessed September 8, 2009).

AHRQ. 2005a. *National hospital available beds for emergencies and disasters (HAvBED) system. Final report and appendixes.* AHRQ Publication No. 05-0103. Rockville: AHRQ.

AHRQ. 2005b. *Altered standards of care in mass casualty events.* AHRQ Publication No. 05-0043. Rockville: AHRQ.

AMA (American Medical Association) Council on Ethical and Judicial Affairs. 1995. Ethical considerations in the allocation of organs and other scarce medical resources among patients. Council on Ethical and Judicial Affairs, American Medical Association. *Arch Intern Med* 155(1):29–40.

AMA. June 2004. *Council on ethical and judicial affairs: Opinion 9.067 - physician obligation in disaster preparedness and response.* http://www.ama-assn.org/ama/pub/physician-resources/medical-ethics/code-medical-ethics/opinion9067.shtml (accessed September 8, 2009).

AMA. 2007. *Basic disaster life support manual, version 2.6.* Chicago: American Medical Association Press.

ANA (American Nurses Association). 2008. *Adapting standards of care under extreme conditions: Guidance for professionals during disasters, pandemics, and other extreme emergencies.* http://www.nursingworld.org/MainMenuCategories/HealthcareandPolicyIssues/DPR/TheLawEthicsofDisasterResponse/AdaptingStandardsofCare.aspx (accessed September 8, 2009).

*93*

Andrulis, D. P., N. J. Siddiqui, and J. L. Gantner. 2007. Preparing racially and ethnically diverse communities for public health emergencies. *Health Aff (Millwood)* 26(5):1269–1279.

ASTHO (The Association of State and Territorial Health Officials). 2009. *At-risk populations guidance document.* http://www.asth.org/Programs/Infectious-Disease/At-Risk-Populations/ (accessed September 8, 2009).

Barbera, J. A., and A. G. MacIntyre. 2007. *Medical surge capacity and capability: A management system for integrating medical and health resources during large-scale emergencies.*2nd edition. Washington, DC: U.S. Department of Health and Human Services.

Barbisch, D. F., and K. L. Koenig. 2006. Understanding surge capacity: Essential elements. *Acad Emerg Med* 13(11):1098–1102.

Beekley, A. C., B. W. Starnes, and J. A. Sebesta. 2007. Lessons learned from modern military surgery. *Surg Clin North Am* 87(1):157–184, vii.

Bernier, R. 2009. *IOM Committee on Guidance for Establishing Standards of Care for Use in Disaster Situations.* Paper presented at IOM Committee on Guidance for Establishing Standards of Care for Use in Disaster Situations, September 2, Washington, DC.

Bernier, R., and E. Marcuse. 2005. *Citizen voices on pandemic flu choices— public engagement pilot project on pandemic influenza.* http://www.hhs.gov/nvpo/PEPPPI/PEPPPICompleteFinalReport.pdf (accessed September 8, 2009).

Berry, P., and M. Matzo. 2004. Death and an aging society. In *Gerontologic palliative care nursing,* edited by M. Matzo and D.W. Sherman. St. Louis, MO: Mosby.

Bierenbaum, A. B., B. Neiley, and C. R. Savageau. 2009. Importance of business continuity in health care. *Disaster Med Public Health Prep* 3(2 Suppl):S7-9.

Binzer, P. 2008. The PREP Act: Liability protection for medical countermeasure development, distribution, and administration. *Biosecur Bioterror* 6(4):293–298.

Burkle, F. M., Jr., E. B. Hsu, M. Loehr, M. D. Christian, D. Markenson, L. Rubinson, and F. L. Archer. 2007. Definition and functions of health unified command and emergency operations centers for large-scale bioevent disasters within the existing ICS. *Disaster Med Public Health Prep* 1(2):135–141.

California Department of Public Health. 2008. *Standards and guidelines for healthcare surge during emergencies.* http://bepreparedcalifornia. ca.gov/EPO/CDPHPrograms/PublicHealthPrograms/EmergencyPrep arednessOffice/EPOProgramsServices/Surge/StandGuide/SSG1.htm (accessed September 8, 2009).

California Emergency Medical Services Authority. 2009. *Disaster Medical Services Division—Hospital Incident Command System (HICS).* http://www.emsa.ca.gov/hics/ (accessed September 4, 2009).

CDC (Centers for Disease Control and Prevention). 2006. *Flusurge 2.0.* http://www.cdc.gov/flu/tools/flusurge/ (accessed September 9, 2009).

CDC. 2009a. *2008–2009 influenza season week 34 ending August 29, 2009.* http://cdc.gov/flu/weekly/index.htm (accessed September 8, 2009).

CDC. 2009b. *Federal public health emergency law: Implications for state and local preparedness and response: Teleconference.* http://www2a.cdc.gov/phlp/webinar_04_29_2009.asp (accessed September 8, 2009).

CDC. 2009c. *Novel H1N1 vaccination recommendations.* http://www. cdc.gov/h1n1flu/vaccination/acip.htm (accessed September 8, 2009).

CDC. 2009d. *Updated interim recommendations for the use of antiviral medications in the treatment and prevention of influenza for the 2009–2010 season.* http://cdc.gov/h1n1flu/recommendations.htm (accessed September 9, 2009).

CDC. 2009e. *Crisis & Emergency Risk Communication (CERC).* http://emergency.cdc.gov/cerc/ (accessed September 8, 2009).

Centers for Law and the Public's Health. 2001. *The model state emergency health powers act (MSEHPA).* http://www.publichealthlaw. net/ModelLaws/MSEHPA.php (accessed September 8, 2009).

Centers for Law and the Public's Health. 2004. *Public health emergency legal preparedness checklist. Civil legal liability and public health emergencies.* Baltimore: Centers for Law and the Public's Health.

Centers for Law and the Public's Health. 2009. *The Model State Emergency Health Powers Act (MSEHPA).* http://www.publichealthlaw. net/ModelLaws/MSEHPA.php (accessed September 8, 2009).

Challen, K., J. Bright, A. Bentley, and D. Walter. 2007. Physiological-social score (PMEWS) vs. CURB-65 to triage pandemic influenza: A comparative validation study using community-acquired pneumonia as a proxy. *BMC Health Serv Res* 7:33.

Hick, J. L., and D. T. O'Laughlin. 2006. Concept of operations for triage of mechanical ventilation in an epidemic. *Acad Emerg Med* 13(2):223–229.

Hick, J. L., L. Rubinson, D. T. O'Laughlin, and J. C. Farmer. 2007. Clinical review: Allocating ventilators during large-scale disasters—problems, planning, and process. *Crit Care* 11(3):217.

Hick, J. L., J. A. Barbera, and G. D. Kelen. 2009. Refining surge capacity: Conventional, contingency, and crisis capacity. *Disaster Med Public Health Prep* 3(2 Suppl):S59–S67.

Hodge, J. G., Jr. 2006. *Emergency System for Advance Registration of Volunteer Health Professionals (ESAR-VHP): Legal and regulatory issues.* Washington, DC: Department of Health and Human Services.

Hodge, J. G., Jr. 2009. The legal landscape for school closures in response to pandemic flu or other public health threats. *Biosecur Bioterror* 7(1):45–50.

Hodge, J., and E. Anderson. 2008. Principles and practice of legal triage during public health emergencies. *NYU Annual Survey of American Law* 64:249–292.

Hodge, J. G., Jr., E. F. Brown, and J. P. O'Connell. 2004. The HIPAA Privacy Rule and bioterrorism planning, prevention, and response. *Biosecur Bioterror* 2(2):73–80.

Hodge, J. G., Jr., E. Anderson, S. P. Teret, J. S. Vernick, T. Kirsch, and G. D. Kelen. 2009a. *Model Memorandum of Understanding between hospitals during declared emergencies.* Baltimore: PACER.

Hodge, J. G., Jr., A. M. Garcia, E. D. Anderson, and T. Kaufman. 2009b. Emergency legal preparedness for hospitals and health care personnel. *Disaster Med Public Health Prep* 3(2 Suppl):S37–S44.

Hoffman, S., R. A. Goodman, and D. D. Stier. 2009. Law, liability, and public health emergencies. *Disaster Med Public Health Prep* 3(2):117–125.

Holt, G. R. 2008. Making difficult ethical decisions in patient care during natural disasters and other mass casualty events. *Otolaryngol Head Neck Surg* 139(2):181–186.

Houston/Harris County Committee on Pandemic Influenza Medical Standards of Care. 2007. *Recommended priority groups for antiviral medication and vaccine.* Houston: Houston Department of Health and Human Services.

IAEA (International Atomic Energy Agency). 2009. *Field triage for mass casualties.* http://www-ns.iaea.org/tech-areas/emergency/iec/tech-areas/emergency/iec/frg/ti9.htm (accessed September 9, 2009).

ICDRM (Institute for Crisis, Disaster, and Risk Management). 2009. *ICDRM/GWU emergency management glossary of terms.* The George Washington University. http://www.gwu.edu/~icdrm/publications/PDF/EM_Glossary_ICDRM.pdf (accessed September 8, 2009).

IOM (Institute of Medicine). 2003. *Preparing for the psychological consequences of terrorism: A public health strategy.* Washington, DC: The National Academies Press. Washington, DC: The National Academies Press.

IOM. 2007. *PTSD compensation and military service.* Washington, DC: The National Academies Press.

IOM. 2008. *Research priorities in emergency preparedness and response for public health systems. A letter report.* Washington, DC: National Academies Press.

IOM. 2009a. *Assessing medical preparedness to respond to a terrorist nuclear event. Workshop report.* Washington, DC: National Academies Press.

IOM. 2009b. *Respiratory protection for healthcare workers in the workplace against novel H1N1 influenza A: A letter report.* Washington, DC: National Academies Press.

IOM. 2009c (unpublished). *Standards of care during a mass casualty event. Workshop summary.* Washington, DC.

Kaji, A., K. L. Koenig, and T. Bey. 2006. Surge capacity for healthcare systems: A conceptual framework. *Acad Emerg Med* 13(11):1157–1159.

Kanter, R. K. 2007. Strategies to improve pediatric disaster surge response: Potential mortality reduction and tradeoffs. *Crit Care Med* 35(12):2837-2842.

Kelen, G. D., C. K. Kraus, M. L. McCarthy, E. Bass, E. B. Hsu, G. Li, J. J. Scheulen, J. B. Shahan, J. D. Brill, and G. B. Green. 2006. Inpatient disposition classification for the creation of hospital surge capacity: A multiphase study. *Lancet* 368(9551):1984–1990.

Kelen, G. D., M. L. McCarthy, C. K. Kraus, R. Ding, E. B. Hsu, G. Li, J. B. Shahan, J. J. Scheulen, and G. B. Green. 2009. Creation of surge capacity by early discharge of hospitalized patients at low risk for untoward events. *Disaster Med Public Health Prep* 3(2 Suppl):S10-16.

Levin, D., Cadigan, R.O., Biddinger, P.D., Condon, S., and H.K. Koh. 2009. Altered Standards of Care During an Influenza Pandemic: Identifying Ethical, Legal, and Practical Principles to Guide Decision Making. *Disaster Medicine and Public Health Preparedness* Epub [published ahead of print].

Lewandowski, W., and K. Adamle. 2009. Substantive areas of clinical nurse specialist practice: A comprehensive review of the literature. *Clin Nurse Spec* 23(2):73-90; quiz 91-72.

Li-Vollmer, M. 2009 September 2, 2009. *IOM Committee on Guidance for Establishing Standards of Care for Use in Disaster Situations.* Paper presented at IOM Committee on Guidance for Establishing Standards of Care for Use in Disaster Situations, September 2, Washington, DC.

Lieberman, D., Nachshon, L., Miloslavsky, O., Dvorkin, V., Shimoni, A., and D. Lieberman. 2009. How do older ventilated patients fare? A survival/functional analysis of 641 ventilations. *Journal of Critical Care* 24(3): 340-46.

Lurie, N., J. Wasserman, and C. D. Nelson. 2006. Public health preparedness: Evolution or revolution? *Health Aff (Millwood)* 25(4):935–945.

Massachusetts Department of Public Health, and Center for Public Health Preparedness at Harvard School of Public Health. 2006 (unpublished). *Planning for altered standards of care during mass casualty events: Scenarios.*

Mastroianni, A. C. 2006. Liability, regulation and policy in surgical innovation: The cutting edge of research and therapy. *Health Matrix Clevel* 16(2):351-442.

Matzo, M. L. 2004. Palliative care: Prognostication and the chronically ill: Methods you need to know as chronic disease progresses in older adults. *Am J Nurs* 104(9):40–49; quiz 50.

McCarthy, M. L., D. Aronsky, and G. D. Kelen. 2006. The measurement of daily surge and its relevance to disaster preparedness. *Acad Emerg Med* 13(11):1138-1141.

McHugh, M., A. B. Staiti, and L. E. Felland. 2004. How prepared are Americans for public health emergencies? Twelve communities weigh in. *Health Aff (Millwood)* 23(3):201–209.

Minnesota Department of Health. 2008. *Minnesota healthcare system preparedness program standards of care for scarce resources.* http//www.health.state.mn.us/oep/healthcare/standards.pdf (accessed September 8, 2009).

Mitchell, S. L., D. K. Kiely, M. B. Hamel, P. S. Park, J. N. Morris, and B. E. Fries. 2004. Estimating prognosis for nursing home residents with advanced dementia. *JAMA* 291(22):2734–2740.

Moreno, R., J. L. Vincent, R. Matos, A. Mendonca, F. Cantraine, L. Thijs, J. Takala, C. Sprung, M. Antonelli, H. Bruining, and S. Willatts. 1999. The use of maximum sofa score to quantify organ dysfunction/failure in intensive care. Results of a prospective, multi-centre study. Working group on sepsis related problems of the esicm. *Intensive Care Med* 25(7):686-696.

National Wildfire Coordinating Group. 1994. *Incident command system national training curriculum instructor guide. Module 16.*

New Jersey Hospital Association. 2008. *Planning today for a pandemic tomorrow: Video vignettes.* http://www.njha.com/paninf/index.aspx (accessed September 8, 2009).

North Central Texas Trauma Regional Advisory Council. 2009. *North Central Texas Trauma Regional Advisory Council hospital mutual aid agreement.* http://ncttrac.org/LinkClick.aspx?fileticket=9N Click.aspx?fileticket=9N6AIZSZ0I4%3D&tabid=66&mid=874 (accessed September 8, 2009).

NYS DOH (New York State Department of Health)/NYS Task Force on Life & the Law. 2007. *Allocation of ventilators in an influenza pandemic:Planning document: Draft for public comment.* http://www.health.state.ny.us/diseases/communicable/influenza/pandemic/ventilators/ (accessed September 8, 2009).

O'Laughlin, D. T., and J. L. Hick. 2008. Ethical issues in resource triage. *Respir Care* 53(2):190–197; discussion 197–200.

Ontario Ministry of Health and Long-term Care. 2008. *Ontario health plan for an influenza pandemic.* http://www.health.gov.on.ca/english/providers/program/emu/pan_flu/pan_flu_plan.html#section (accessed September 8, 2009).

Pastor, M., R. Bullard, J. Boyce, A. Fothergill, R. Morello-Frosch, and B. Wright. 2006. *Report: In the wake of the storm: Environment, disaster, and race after Katrina.* New York, NY: Russell Sage Foundation

Pegalis, S. 2009. Physician and surgeon liability: Standard of care, generally. *American Law of Medical Malpractice* 3(3).

Peres Bota, D., C. Melot, F. Lopes Ferreira, V. Nguyen Ba, and J. L. Vincent. 2002. The multiple organ dysfunction score (MODS) versus the sequential organ failure assessment (SOFA) score in outcome prediction. *Intensive Care Med* 28(11):1619-1624.

Pesik, N., M. E. Keim, and K. V. Iserson. 2001. Terrorism and the ethics of emergency medical care. *Ann Emerg Med* 37(6):642–646.

Pettila, V., M. Pettila, S. Sarna, P. Voutilainen, and O. Takkunen. 2002. Comparison of multiple organ dysfunction scores in the prediction of hospital mortality in the critically ill. *Crit Care Med* 30(8):1705-1711.

Phillips, S., and A. Knebel, eds. 2007. *Mass medical care with scarce resources: A community planning guide.* AHRQ Publication No. 07-0001. Rockville: AHRQ.

Pollack, M. M., U. E. Ruttimann, and P. R. Getson. 1988. Pediatric Risk of Mortality (PRISM) score. *Crit Care Med* 16(11):1110–1116.

Posner, Z., H. Admi, and N. Menashe. 2003. Ten-fold expansion of a burn unit in mass casualty: How to recruit the nursing staff. *Disaster Manag Response* 1(4):100–104.

Powell, T., K. C. Christ, and G. S. Birkhead. 2008. Allocation of ventilators in a public health disaster. *Disaster Med Public Health Prep* 2(1):20–26.

Propper, B. W., T. E. Rasmussen, S. B. Davidson, S. L. Vandenberg, W. D. Clouse, G. E. Burkhardt, S. M. Gifford, and J. A. Johannigman. 2009. Surgical response to multiple casualty incidents following single explosive events. *Ann Surg* 250(2):311–315.

REMM. 2009. *REMM triage guidelines.* http://www.remm.nlm.gov/radtriage.htm (accessed September 9, 2009).

Romig, L. 2009. *The jumpstart pediatric mci triage tool.* http://www.jumpstarttriage.com/ (accessed August 31, 2009).

Rosenbaum, S., M. B. Harty, and J. Sheer. 2008. State laws extending comprehensive legal liability protections for professional health-care volunteers during public health emergencies. *Public Health Rep* 123(2):238–241.

Rubinson, L., J. B. Nuzzo, D. S. Talmor, T. O'Toole, B. R. Kramer, and T. V. Inglesby. 2005. Augmentation of hospital critical care capacity after bioterrorist attacks or epidemics: Recommendations of the working group on emergency mass critical care. *Crit Care Med* 33(10):2393-2403.

Rubinson, L., J. L. Hick, D. G. Hanfling, A. V. Devereaux, J. R. Dichter, M. D. Christian, D. Talmor, J. Medina, J. R. Curtis, and J. A. Geiling. 2008. Definitive care for the critically ill during a disaster: A framework for optimizing critical care surge capacity: From a task force for mass critical care summit meeting, January 26–27, 2007, Chicago, IL. *Chest* 133(5 Suppl):18S–31S.

Saffle, J. R., N. Gibran, and M. Jordan. 2005. Defining the ratio of outcomes to resources for triage of burn patients in mass casualties. *J Burn Care Rehabil* 26(6):478–482.

Schmidt, P. J. 2002. Blood and disaster-supply and demand. *N Engl J Med* 346(8):617–620.

Schoch-Spana, M., C. Franco, J. B. Nuzzo, and C. Usenza. 2007. Community engagement: Leadership tool for catastrophic health events. *Biosecur Bioterror* 5(1):8–25.

Schreiber, M. 2005. *Learning from 9/11: Toward a national model for children and families in mass casualty. In on the ground after 9/11: Mental health responses and practical knowledge gained.* Edited by Y. Daneili. New York, NY: Haworth.

Schultz, C. H., and K. L. Koenig. 2006. State of research in high-consequence hospital surge capacity. *Acad Emerg Med* 13(11):1153-1156.

Sharpe, V. A. 2009. *IOM Committee on Guidance for Establishing Standards of Care for Use in Disaster Situations.* Paper presented at IOM Committee on Guidance for Establishing Standards of Care for Use in Disaster Situations, September 2, Washington, DC.

Sheppard, B., G. J. Rubin, J. K. Wardman, and S. Wessely. 2006. Terrorism and dispelling the myth of a panic prone public. *J Public Health Policy* 27(3):219-245; discussion 246-219.

Skidmore, S., W. Wall, and J. Church. 2003. *Modular emergency medical system concept of operation for the acute care center: Mass casualty strategy for a biological terror incident.* Department of Defense.

State of Connecticut. 2006. *State of connecticut emergency management hospital mutual aid agreement.* http://www.ynhhs.org/emergency/commu/OEP_Emergency_Management_MOU.pdf (accessed September 8, 2009).

Stein-Spencer, L. 2009. *IOM Committee on Guidance for Establishing Standards of Care for Use in Disaster Situations.* Paper presented at IOM Committee on Guidance for Establishing Standards of Care for Use in Disaster Situations, September 2, Washington, DC.

Stier, D. 2009. *Public health law program: Mutual aid.* http://www2a.cdc.gov/phlp/mutualaid/ (accessed August 31, 2009).

Swendiman, K. S., and N. L. Jones. 2009. *The 2009 influenza pandemic: Selected legal issues.* Washington, DC: Congressional Research Services.

Tabery, J., and C. W. Mackett, 3rd. 2008. Ethics of triage in the event of an influenza pandemic. *Disaster Med Public Health Prep* 2(2):114–118.

Talmor, D., A. E. Jones, L. Rubinson, M. D. Howell, and N. I. Shapiro. 2007. Simple triage scoring system predicting death and the need for critical care resources for use during epidemics. *Crit Care Med* 35(5):1251–1256.

TFAH (Trust for America's Health). 2008. TFAH liability protections: relevant statutes. http://healthyamericans.org/reports/bioterror08/pdf/legal-preparedness-law-review-of-state-statutes-and-codes.pdf (accessed September 11, 2009).

The Commonwealth of Massachusetts Department of Public Health. May 2007 (unpublished). *Guidelines for the development of altered standards of care for influenza pandemic.*

The Sphere Project. 2004. *Humanitarian charter and minimum standards in disaster response.* Oxford: Oxfam Publishing.

The Utah Hospitals and Health Systems Association. 2009. *Utah pandemic influenza hospital and ICU triage guidelines. Version 1.* http://www.pandemicflu.utah.gov/plan/med_triage011009.pdf (accessed September 8, 2009).

Thienkrua, W., B. L. Cardozo, M. L. Chakkraband, T. E. Guadamuz, W. Pengjuntr, P. Tantipiwatanaskul, S. Sakornsatian, S. Ekassawin, B. Panyayong, A. Varangrat, J. W. Tappero, M. Schreiber, and F. van Griensven. 2006. Symptoms of posttraumatic stress disorder and depression among children in tsunami-affected areas in southern Thailand. *JAMA* 296(5):549–559.

Toner, E., R. Waldhorn, C. Franco, B. Courtney, K. Rambhia, A. Norwood, T. Inglesby, and T. O'Toole. 2009. *Hospitals rising to the challenge: The first five years of the U.S. hospital preparedness program and priorities going forward.* Baltimore: Center for Biosecurity of UPMC.

Townsend, F. 2006. *The federal response to Hurricane Katrina: Lessons learned.* http://georgewbush-whitehouse.archives.gov/reports/katrina-lessons-learned/ (accessed September 8, 2009).

University of California–Davis, and C. E. Sandrock. 2009 (unpublished). *ESCAPE partnership crisis care guidelines.* http://www.ucdmc.ucdavis.edu/escape/crisis-care-guidelines.html (accessed September 8, 2009).

University of Toronto. 2005. *Stand on guard for thee: Ethical considerations in preparedness planning for pandemic influenza.* University of Toronto Joint Centre for Bioethics Pandemic Influenza Working Group. Toronto: University of Toronto.

VHA (Veterans Health Administration). 2008 (unpublished). *Tertiary triage protocol for allocation of scarce life-saving resources in VHA during an influenza pandemic.* http://www.ethics.va.gov/docs/pandemicflu/Draft_VHA_Pan_Flu_Tertiary_Triage_Protocol_20090427.doc (accessed September 8, 2009).

VHA. 2009 (unpublished). *Draft guidance: Meeting the challenge of pandemic influenza: Ethical guidance for VHA leaders and clinicians.* http://www.ethics.va.gov/activities/pandemic_influenza_preparedness.asp (accessed September 8, 2009).

Vincent, J. L., A. de Mendonca, F. Cantraine, R. Moreno, J. Takala, P. M. Suter, C. L. Sprung, F. Colardyn, and S. Blecher. 1998. Use of the sofa score to assess the incidence of organ dysfunction/failure in intensive care units: Results of a multicenter, prospective study. Working group on "Sepsis-related problems" Of the european society of intensive care medicine. *Crit Care Med* 26(11):1793-1800.

Vincent, J. L., R. Moreno, J. Takala, S. Willatts, A. De Mendonca, H. Bruining, C. K. Reinhart, P. M. Suter, and L. G. Thijs. 1996. The sofa (sepsis-related organ failure assessment) score to describe organ dysfunction/failure. On behalf of the working group on sepsis-related problems of the european society of intensive care medicine. *Intensive Care Med* 22(7):707-710.

Virginia Department of Health. 2008. *Virginia Hospital and Healthcare Association Altered Standards of Care Workgroup: Critical resource shortages: A planning guide.* http://www.troutmansanders.com/files/

upload/Critical%20Resource%20Shortages-A%20Planning%20Guid
e.pdf (accessed September 8, 2009).

Walter, L. C., R. J. Brand, S. R. Counsell, R. M. Palmer, C. S. Landefeld,
R. H. Fortinsky, and K. E. Covinsky. 2001. Development and validation of a prognostic index for 1-year mortality in older adults after
hospitalization. *JAMA* 285(23):2987–2994.

Washington State Department of Health's Altered Standards of Care
Workgroup. October 2008 (unpublished). *Report and recommendations to the department of health secretary on establishing altered
standards of care during an influenza pandemic.*

Waselenko, J. K., T. J. MacVittie, W. F. Blakely, N. Pesik, A. L. Wiley,
W. E. Dickerson, H. Tsu, D. L. Confer, C. N. Coleman, T. Seed,
P. Lowry, J. O. Armitage, and N. Dainiak. 2004. Medical management of the acute radiation syndrome: Recommendations of the Strategic National Stockpile Radiation Working Group. *Ann Intern Med*
140(12):1037–1051.

White, D. B., M. H. Katz, J. M. Luce, and B. Lo. 2009. Who should receive life support during a public health emergency? Using ethical
principles to improve allocation decisions. *Ann Intern Med*
150(2):132–138.

WHO (World Health Organization). 2006. *Project on addressing ethical
issues in pandemic influenza planning: Equitable access to therapeutic and prophylactic measures.* http://www.who.int/eth/ethics/PIE
thicsdraftpaperWG12oct06.pdf (accessed September 8, 2009).

WHO. 2008. *Closing the gap in a generation: Health equity through action on the social determinants of health. Final report of the Commission on Social Determinants of Health.* Geneva: WHO.

WHO. 2009a. *Project on addressing ethical issues in pandemic influenza
planning: Equitable access to therapeutic and prophylactic measures.* http://www.who.int/eth/ethics/PIEthicsdraftpaperWG12oct06.
pdf (accessed September 8, 2009).

WHO. 2009b. *Pandemic (H1N1) 2009— update 62 (revised 21 August
2009).* http://www.who.int/csr/don/2009_08_21/en/index.html
(accessed September 8, 2009).

Wilkinson, A., and M. Matzo. 2006. *Palliative care and mass casualty
events in rendering mass medical care with scarce resources: A
planning guide.* Rockville: AHRQ.

Wynia, M. 2005. Oversimplifications I: Physicians don't do public
health. *Am J Bioeth* 5(4):4-5.

Wynia, M. 2009. *IOM Committee on Guidance for Establishing Standards of Care for Use in Disaster Situations*. Paper presented at IOM Committee on Guidance for Establishing Standards of Care for Use in Disaster Situations, September 2, Washington, DC.

# B

# Glossary

Alternate care facility

A temporary site that is not located on hospital property, established to provide patient care. It may provide either ambulatory or non-ambulatory care. It may serve to "decompress" hospitals that are maximally filled, or to bolster community-based triage capabilities. Has also been referred to as an "alternate care site."

Clinical care committee

Composed of clinical and administrative leaders at a healthcare institution, this committee is responsible for making prioritization decisions about the allocation of critical life-sustaining interventions. The clinical care committee may also be formed at the healthcare coalition level (e.g., hospital, primary care, emergency medical services agency, public health, emergency management. and others), playing the role of the disaster medical advisory committee at the regional level (see disaster medical advisory committee). May appoint a triage team (see triage team) to evaluate case-by-case decisions.

Contingency surge

The spaces, staff, and supplies used are not consistent with daily practices, but provide care that is *functionally equivalent* to usual patient care practices. These spaces or practices may be used temporarily during a major mass casualty incident or on a more sustained basis during a disaster (when the demands of the incident exceed community resources) (Hick et al., 2009).

Conventional capacity

The spaces, staff, and supplies used are consistent with daily practices within the institution. These spaces and practices are used during a major mass casualty incident that triggers activation of the facility emergency operations plan (Hick et al., 2009).

Crisis standards of care

The level of care possible during a crisis or disaster due to limitations in supplies, staff, environment, or other factors. These standards will usually incorporate the following principles: (1) prioritize population health rather than individual outcomes; (2) respect ethical principles of beneficence, stewardship, equity, and trust; (3) modify regulatory requirements to provide liability protection for healthcare providers making resource allocation decisions; and/or (4) designate a crisis triage officer and include provisions for palliative care in triage models for scarce resource allocation (e.g., ventilators) (Chang et al., 2008). Crisis standards of care will usually follow a formal declaration or recognition by state government during a pervasive (pandemic influenza) or catastrophic (earthquake, hurricane) disaster which recognizes that contingency surge response strategies (resource-sparing strategies) have been exhausted, and crisis medical care must be provided for a sustained period of time. Formal recognition of these austere operating conditions enables specific legal/regulatory powers and protections for healthcare provider allocation of scarce medical resources and for alternate care facility operations. Under these conditions, the goal is still to supply the best care possible to each patient.

Crisis surge

Adaptive spaces, staff, and supplies are not consistent with usual standards of care, but provide sufficiency of care in the setting of a catastrophic disaster (i.e., provide the best possible care to patients given the circumstances and resources available). Crisis capacity activation constitutes a *significant* adjustment to standards of care (Hick et al., 2009).

Disaster medical advisory committee

At the state or regional level, evaluates evidence-based, peer-reviewed critical care and other decision tools and recommends decision-making algorithms to be used when life-sustaining resources become scarce. May also be involved in providing broader recommendations regarding disaster planning and response efforts. When formed at the regional level, this group may take on the same functions as that of the clinical care committee. Those functions are focused in two distinct areas—medical advisory input and resource allocation decision approval.

| Emergency response system | A formal or informal organization covering a specified geographic area minimally composed of healthcare institutions, public health agencies, emergency management agencies, and emergency medical service providers to facilitate regional preparedness planning and response. |
|---|---|
| EMS (emergency medical services/system) | A system of healthcare professionals, facilities, and equipment providing out-of-hospital emergency care. |
| Healthcare coalition | A group of individual healthcare assets (e.g., hospitals, clinics, long-term care facilities, etc.) in a specified geographic location that have partnered to respond to emergencies in a coordinated manner. The coalition has both a preparedness element and a response organization that possess appropriate structures, processes, and procedures. During response, the goals of the coalition are to facilitate situational awareness, resource support, and coordination of incident management among the participating organizations (ICDRM, 2009). |
| Healthcare institution | Any facility providing patient care. This includes acute care hospitals, community health centers, long-term care institutions, private practices, and skilled nursing facilities. |
| Healthcare practitioners | Includes "healthcare professionals" and other non-licensed individuals who are involved in the delivery of healthcare services. |

Healthcare professionals

Individuals who are licensed to provide healthcare services under state law.

Indicator

Measurement or predictor that is used to recognize surge capacity and capability problems within the healthcare system, suggesting that crisis standards of care may become necessary and requiring further analysis or system actions to prevent overload.

Legal standard of care

The minimum amount of care and skill that a healthcare practitioner must exercise in particular circumstances based on what a reasonable and prudent healthcare practitioner would do in similar circumstances; during non-emergencies and disasters, they are based on the specific situation.

Medical standard of care

The type and level of medical care required by professional norms, professional requirements, and institutional objectives; these standards vary as circumstances change, including during emergencies or crisis events.

Memorandums of Understanding (MOUs)

A voluntary agreement among agencies cies and/or jurisdictions for the purpose of providing mutual aid at the time of a disaster.

Mutual aid agreements (MAAs)

Written instrument between agencies and/or jurisdictions in which they agree to assist one another on request by furnishing personnel and equipment. An "agreement" is generally more legally binding than an "understanding" (Barbera and Macintyre, 2007).

Palliative care

Medical care provided by an interdisciplinary team to prevent and relieve suffering and to support the best possible quality of life for patients and their families, regardless of the stage of the disease or the need for other therapies. Palliative care affirms life by supporting the patient and family's goals for the future, including their hopes for cure or life prolongation, as well as their hopes for peace and dignity throughout the course of illness, the dying process, and death.

Protocol

A written procedural approach to a specific problem or condition.

Public health system

A complex network of individuals, organizations, and relevant critical infrastructures that have the potential to act individually and together to create conditions of health, including communities, healthcare delivery systems (e.g., home care, ambulatory care, private practice, hospitals, skilled nursing facilities, and others), employers and business, the media, homeland security and public safety, academia, and the governmental public health infrastructure (IOM, 2008).

Resource sparing

The process of maximizing the utility of supplies and material through conservation, substitution, reuse, adaptation, and reallocation.

Scope of practice

The extent of a professional's ability to provide health services pursuant to their competence and license, certification, privileges, or other lawful authority to practice.

SOFA score

The Sequential Organ Failure Assessment (SOFA) score is a scoring system to determine the extent of a person's organ function or rate of failure. The score is based on six different body systems: respiratory, cardiovascular, hepatic, hematopoietic, renal, and neurologic.

Triage

The process of sorting patients and allocating aid on the basis of need for or likely benefit from medical treatment. Several types of triage are referenced in this letter:

- Primary triage: The first triage of patients into the medical system (it may occur out of hospital), at which point patients are assigned an acuity level based on the severity of their illness/disease.
- Secondary triage: Reevaluation of the patient's condition after initial medical care. This may occur at the hospital following EMS interventions or after initial interventions in the emergency department. This often involves the decision to admit the patient to the hospital.
- Tertiary triage: Further reevaluation of the patients' response to treatment after further interventions; this is ongoing during their hospital stay. This is the least practiced and least well-defined type of triage.

Triage team

Appointed by the clinical care committee, uses decision tools appropriate to the event and resource being triaged, making tertiary triage using scarce resource allocation decisions. This is similar in concept to triage teams established to evaluate incoming patients to the emergency department requiring primary or secondary triage, usually in a sudden-onset, no-notice disaster event (e.g., explosive detonation).

Trigger

Evidence that austere conditions prevail so that crisis standard of care practices will be required. This may occur at an institutional, and often regional, level of response. It suggests the need for the immediate implementation of response pathways that are required to manage a crisis surge response emanating from the disaster situation.

# C

# Crisis Standards of Care
# Implementation Guidance Scenarios

Applying the guidance and principles laid out in the report, the committee developed two brief case studies that may serve to illustrate the implementation crisis standards of care. Recognizing the current attention and concern around the 2009 influenza A (H1N1) pandemic, one scenario focuses on a gradual-onset pandemic flu modeled around potential issues that may arise this upcoming flu season. The second scenario focuses on the issues that would arise due to a no-notice, sudden-onset event, and uses a devastating earthquake event as the model. For each scenario specific activities are indicated in italics and mapped by number to key elements and core components from the committee's guidance.

## Major Influenza Pandemic Scenario

**Key elements/core components**

**Scenario Description:** An influenza pandemic was selected to demonstrate a response to the need to implement crisis standards of care as a result of a gradual-onset disaster event. This scenario is based on response to an infectious agent of high transmissibility and low pathogenicity with greater impact on younger age groups.

**Scenario:**
Preevent Planning:
    In anticipation of a possible severe influenza pandemic, the state health department convened a *multidisciplinary group composed₁* of ethics, medical, legal, public health, emergency management, and emergency management services

₁State Public Authority Process:
Guideline development group

(EMS) experts and members of the public (represented by key faith, cultural, and at-risk group representatives) to provide advice on pandemic preparedness. This group suggested enabling legislation for declaring a public health emergency, improving liability protection during disasters for volunteer and non-volunteer healthcare providers, and expanding the scope of practice for many healthcare providers. A smaller *medical advisory committee$_2$* of critical care, infectious disease, emergency, and pediatric physicians developed draft guidelines dealing with potential alterations in the healthcare system during the time of a pandemic. These guidelines dealt with alteration in standards of care to crisis standards of care, if necessary, during a pandemic, addressing issues such as intensive care unit (ICU) admission criteria using Sequential Organ Failure Assessment (SOFA) scoring and ventilator allocation based on work done in New York and Minneapolis. These guidelines were carefully reviewed by the larger advisory committee with state-wide provider and community engagement and incorporated the *ethical principles$_3$* of fairness, duty to care, duty to steward resources, transparency, consistency across institutions and accountability. This group also established *indicators$_4$* (ICU bed availability, ventilator availability, emergency department [ED] average wait times) to follow on regional and state levels to assist in the monitoring of disease progression and status, which were already tracked by a *state-wide EMS and hospital monitoring system$_5$*. The Disaster Medical Advisory Committee was tasked with obtaining quarterly data from this system and determining thresholds that would prompt an alert to the regional hospital coalition that patient care demand for services was increasing. State preparation also included planning for the establishment of alternate care facilities, if necessary, for acute, palliative, and behavioral health care. Purchases of antiviral medications, N95 masks, materials to provide care at an alternate care site, and a small number of ventilators were purchased using federal grant funding as well as a state legislative appropriation.

$_2$State Public Authority Process: State Disaster Medical Advisory Committee

$_3$Ethical Elements: Core ethical components listed

$_4$Indicators and Triggers: Event-specific resource availability

$_5$Indicators and Triggers: Situational awareness monitoring

The Event:

In early fall, a novel influenza virus was detected in the United States. Cases rapidly spread across pockets of the United States. The virus exhibited a mortality rate double the usual expected influenza mortality, with a predilection toward school-age children. Emergency departments across the state began to see a marked rise in patient volumes, and concerns were expressed that resources required for the sustained delivery of patient care might be strained. The state *disaster medical advisory committee*[6] was convened, with supplemental representation from pediatric and pediatric critical care in addition to the committee's usual representatives. The committee made revisions to their prior guidance to manage a surge in patient care demand based on available epidemiologic information. *Information was circulated to clinicians and nursing personnel*[7] reminding them of the planning work and several interviews and television news features were used as an opportunity to reinforce hopeful, yet realistic *messaging about preparedness*[8] for a possible scarce resource situation. The state Department of Health (DOH) opened their *Department Operations Center*[9] to monitor the situation, passing along updates from the Centers for Disease Control and Prevention (CDC) and other partners as needed. The State Disaster Medical Advisory Committee (SDMAC) worked with DOH staff to develop and vet outpatient screening tools. A few of the in-state regional hospital coalitions convened their own *regional advisory committees*[10] to modify and customize this guidance to make it applicable for their local needs. At the hospital level, pandemic planning included members of the predesignated disaster *clinical care committees*[11], who approved and/or modified these tools and guidance for institutional use. As the pandemic increased in intensity, state and regional advisory committee members updated contact information and participated in weekly conference calls.

*Monitoring*[12] of hospital ICU occupancy, hospital divert status, healthcare provider absenteeism, and business closures demonstrated a worsening situation in the state in late October. The state requested activation of the Strategic National Stockpile (SNS) for delivery of additional antiviral medications and personal protective equipment

[6] State Public Authority Process: Event-based use of State Disaster Medical Advisory Committee

[7] Incident Management – State Role; Community and Provider Engagement: Stakeholder roles and involvement

[8] Crisis Standards of Care Operations: Use of Regional Disaster Medical Advisory Committee

[9] Department Operations Center

[10] Incident management – State Agency Role

[11] Clinical Process and Operations: Clinical care in crisis situations

[12] Indicators and Triggers: Situational awareness

[13]Legal Authority and Environment: mutual aid agreements; Crisis standard of care operations: Use of the Regional Medical Coordinating Center (RMCC)

[14]State Public Authorities Process: Public health emergency

[15]Clinical Process and Operations: Communications strategies

[16]Clinical Process and operations: Resource-sparing strategies

[17]Community and Provider engagement: Crisis risk communications

[18]Clinical Process and Operations: Incident management principles

[19]Clinical Process and Operations: Intrastate regional consistency

[20]Legal Authority and Environment: State declaration of public health emergency

[21]Legal Authority and Environment: Licensing and credentialing

(PPE). The state's emergency operations center (EOC) was opened and *interfacility Memorandums of Understanding*[13] were activated. The State DOH coordination efforts relocated to the state EOC. Area hospitals moved from conventional care to contingency care as the pandemic worsened, with many reducing elective surgeries, boarding ICU patients in stepdown units, boarding floor patients in procedure and postanesthesia care areas, and *setting up rapid screening and treatment areas*[14] for the mildly ill apart from the emergency department, where volumes had escalated to nearly double usual daily volumes. Homecare agencies noted a significant increase in the acuity and volume of their patient referrals. Ambulatory care clinics had to clear schedules to accommodate the volume of acute illness, *despite media messages*[15] to stay home unless severely ill and it was difficult reaching clinics because there phone lines were tied up much of the time. Hospitals activated their *Hospital Incident Command System*[16], using action planning cycles and providing daily updates to staff. The Regional Medical Coordinating Center (RMCC) for the local hospital coalition of 24 hospitals was stood up and provided *situational awareness*[17] and acted as the liaison among hospitals and public health, EMS, and emergency management. Conference calls became daily, and a web-based information sharing system was also used to post guidelines, talking points, and other information and issues.

State-wide, a *public health emergency*[18] was declared by the governor. This declaration allowed for the temporary adaptation of certain *licensing, medical supervision, and credentialing regulations*[19]. More generous nurse-patient ratios were also allowed. Alternate care facilities were opened, initially to provide early treatment to those with minor illness, but as the situation worsened, the RMCC worked with public health and EMS agencies to *broaden the scope of care*[20] to include intravenous fluid hydration, and EMS was allowed to transport patients directly to these centers. The SDMAC participated in several conference calls with RMCC and regional medical *advisors to facilitate and provide ideas on care provision and staffing*[21], as these functions were not included in the initial planning for "flu centers".

Hospital and EMS staffing requirements were waived by the governor. The Secretary of Health and Human Services issued a *waiver of sanctions*[22] for noncompliance with certain EMTALA requirements. The state Department of Health (DOH) engaged in aggressive risk communication to try to reduce patients with mild illness presenting to clinics or EDs, taking care that its messages were consistent with those provided by the CDC.

The state DOH requested that the RMCCs submit their *incident action plans (IAPs)*[23] on a consistent 8am cycle, and these were reviewed and summarized within the state IAP at 10am. Occasional discrepancies in medical care decision making was noted in review of the regional IAPs. Those that demonstrated a significant *lack of consistency*[24] were discussed with the chair of the SDMAC, and as needed with the full committee, and then were *addressed with the region*[25].

As demand increased, hospital incident commanders convened their *clinical care committees*[26] in order to prioritize available hospital resources toward patient care, as well as anticipating those resources that may soon be in short supply. Many of these committees used prior guidance for scarce resource situations from the state DOH and other "evidence-based" sources in their recommendations at each operational period *to the incident commander*[27]. ICU capacity was generally spilling over to monitored units, with stable patients from floor beds being *transferred to alternate care sites or sent home with homecare*[28]. Ventilators were now noted to be in extremely short supply. The clinical care committees reviewed triage processes recommended by the state and assured that staff and policies were prepared in case ventilator *triage was required*[29].

Based on the worsening situation, and state DOH estimates that ventilator triage would be required at any time, the governor issued an *executive order*[30] recognizing a "crisis standard of care" and providing legal protections to healthcare workers who were responding according to existing plans in a good-faith manner. The state DOH formally issued ventilator *triage guidance*[31] as well as guidance on conservation of oxygen use which had been previously recommended and approved as a *resource-sparing strategy*[32] by the SDMAC and guideline advisory group. The SDMAC met by

[22] Legal Authority and Environment: Scopes of practice for healthcare professionals

[23] Legal Authority and Environment: Special emergency protections

[24] Clinical Process and Operations: Healthcare facility responsibilities – clinical care committee

[25] Legal Authorities: Executive order

[26] Clinical Process and Operations: Intrastate regional consistencies

[27] Clinical Process and Operations: Communications strategies

[28] Clinical Process and Operations: Coordination of resource management

[29] Clinical Process and Operations: Coordination extends through all elements of health system

[30] Clinical Process and Operations: Application of decision support tools and triage teams; Legal Authority and Environment: Medical and legal standards of care

[31] Clinical Process and Operations: Application of decision support tools

[32] Clinical Process and Operations: Resource-sparing strategies

conference call frequently to discuss possible updates to the guidance, but the epidemiology of the disease did not allow for incorporation of further prognostic indicators based on the specific epidemic virus.

As conditions continued to deteriorate, some reports of public unrest were noted. Tempers ran high as wait times in private physician offices, ambulatory clinics and hospital emergency departments lengthened. Community leaders issued *messages[33]* via the local print and broadcast media reiterating the extensive health and medical response planning that had already been conducted, as well as a description of those plans presently under consideration, including the possibility that resources may become in exceedingly short supply.

[33]Community and Provider Engagement: Community trust and assurance

The situation was worsening. Institutional surge capacity was exceeded, especially by pediatric patients, with many hospitals having to move to crisis care with implementation of ICU triage criteria and ventilator allocation. *"Triage teams[34]"* were thus activated to assist with these clinical allocation decisions by their institutional clinical care committees. Rural hospitals used a phone-in metropolitan hospital triage team (three were set up in the state via the RMCC in coordination with state DOH) when a patient in respiratory failure presented to their facility – if the patient qualified for a ventilation trial, the metro team arranged for transfer to a tertiary center. Such calls were few, however, as all *hospitals had an understanding[35]* of the types of patients eligible for ventilation trials based on daily conference calls hosted by the RMCC (in which the state DOH participated in) and the Internet communication system used by that hospital coalition.

[34]State Public Authority Process: Triage teams

[35]Clinical Process and Operations: Communications strategies

[36]Clinical Process and Operations: Inclusion of palliative care principles

*Palliative care[36]* areas were designated in several facilities and were set up in a hotel in one case. The RMCC requested operational guidance for that facility from the SDMAC, which worked with preidentified subject-matter experts to create printed guidance and recommendations for this novel operation, which was then *shared with all the hospitals[37]* in the state. Slowly, intensive care admits began to decline, and the triage team was

[37]Clinical Process and Operations: Intrastate regional consistencies

[38]Clinical Process and
Operations: Mental health needs

disbanded, though the clinical care committee was required to supervise phased transition back through contingency and crisis care. After 7 weeks, the pandemic began to abate, and clinical care returned to conventional status, though the work of behavioral health practitioners had just begun. Patients with *mental health needs*[38] continued to stress many elements of the healthcare delivery system and required significant resources. Alternate care sites that were once used as "flu centers" or to help decompress overwhelmed hospitals were now being used to provide mental health screening and therapeutics, when indicated. This aspect of the recovery phase would continue to tax healthcare workers and the public at large for many weeks, as many patients who had deferred their usual or chronic care during the pandemic now presented to clinics and emergency departments.

[39]Community and Provider
Engagement: Community
cultural values and boundaries;
Continuity of community
education and awareness

The state DOH and SDMAC prepared after-action reports which were reviewed by the broader guideline advisory group and a larger group of medical stakeholders prior to their release to the RMCCs and public. The guideline advisory group and state DOH also hosted *hearings in each of the regions*[39] to allow public and provider input, as well as making an anonymous online system available for comments in order to improve response for future events.

# Major Earthquake Scenario

**Key elements/core components**

**Scenario Description:** A major earthquake scenario was selected to demonstrate the need to implement crisis standards of care as a result of a catastrophic, sudden onset disaster event. This scenario is based on response to a devastating disaster event that is regional in scope. However, it highlights many of the basic key elements and core components required to implement crisis standards of care in a disaster.

**Scenario:**

It is a relatively quiet afternoon in the emergency department of Hillendale Hospital in Southern California, a 232-bed Level 2 trauma center, when without warning, the shaking begins. Personnel respond quickly to protect patients according to emergency plans.

A magnitude 7.8 earthquake has occurred on the southernmost 300 km (200 mi) of the San Andreas Fault, between the Salton Sea and Lake Hughes, California. The sudden rupture of this fault produced very strong shaking near the fault line, with medium to long durations. Along with the initial shaking came liquefaction and devastating landslides.

[1] Clinical Process and Operations: Incident management principles

[2] Clinical Process and Operations: Coordination of resource management

[3] Indicators and Triggers: Situational awareness and management

[4] Indicators and Triggers: Critical infrastructure disruption

After the initial shaking stops, the nursing supervisor *activates the hospital emergency operations plan*[1] and assumes the initial incident command role under the Hospital Incident Command System (HICS). The emergency operations center is opened and *callbacks to staff*[2] are attempted. An initial damage survey is conducted by facility engineers and reveals that the hospital has numerous critical mission functions that are disrupted. The hospital campus is reliant on generator power. Water pressure is dangerously low. There is no major structural damage to the facility, however. Based on *radio reports and "tweets" through the online service Twitter*[3], this major quake has shut down main highways and roads across the area to the south, disrupted cellular phone and landline phone service, and left *most of the area without power*[4]. Several fires are burning out of control in the metropolitan area about 12 miles south of the hospital.

Within 20 minutes after the quake, a steady stream of those with minor injuries and occasional major trauma begin arriving. The walking wounded are triaged to the cafeteria and provided first aid. The emergency room begins to fill with more seriously wounded who are moved upstairs to beds as quickly as possible. As usual, the hospital was fairly full, but a procedure area has been converted to patient care. Surgeons take several cases to the operating room, performing bailout procedures in order to free staff and space for subsequently arriving cases. Due to the power outage, *no elective cases are being performed*[5].

5Clinical Process and Operations: Resource-sparing strategies

6Clinical Process and Operations: Coordination of resource management, use of clinical care committee

7Clinical Process and Operations: Resource-sparing strategies; Ethical Elements: Duty to steward resources

A few staff are able to make it in to the hospital, including an administrator who takes over the role of incident commander and requests that the nursing supervisor pull together members of the predetermined clinical care committee in order to *take stock of available resources*[6] and, in conjunction with the planning chief, *determine ways to conserve*[7] blood products, intravenous fluids, narcotics, antibiotics, and surgical supplies. The hospital administrator assumes that resupply of these key resources is unlikely for the next few days. Fortunately, the hospital has prepared well for food, water, and utilities disruption and can safely continue to operate for now.

8Clinical Care and Operations: use of the Regional Medical Coordination Center

The Regional Medical Coordination Center (RMCC) for Hillendale's hospital coalition has been established now at the back-up *jurisdictional emergency operations center (EOC)*[8]. This is because the primary EOC has been heavily damaged due to fire. Hillendale requests assistance to provide patient care and advises that they will need fuel, water and supplies within a few days, but several other regional *hospitals have been more heavily damaged*[9], and their requests take priority. The RMCC notes that a common challenge for hospital response is the lack of blood products and intravenous fluids sufficient to treat crush injuries. Patients requiring regularly scheduled dialysis are also an issue, as are patients with home ventilators that lack power. Finally, with resupply of hospital liquid oxygen in doubt, questions of conservation arise. The *RMCC works with public health*[10] to identify resources for the home ventilator

9Indicators and Triggers: Disruption of social and community functioning

10Legal Authority and Environment: Mutual aid agreements

[11]Clinical Process and Operations: State Disaster Medical Advisory Committee

[12]Legal Authority and Environment: Scope of practice

[13]Clinical Process and Operations: Communications strategies

[14]Clinical Process and Operations: Incident management—jurisdiction

[15]Clinical Operations and Process: Incident management—state and federal

[16]Indicators and Triggers: Situational awareness

[17]Clinical Process and Operations: Coordination extends through all elements of health system

[18]Indicators and Triggers: Disruption of community functioning

[19]Community and Provider Engagement: Provider roles and involvement

[20]Clinical Process and Operations: Resource-sparing strategies

population, and the RMCC contacts the state Department of Health (DOH) about the other issues – the state DOH posts prepared guidance on dialysis patients and blood products which has previously been developed by *the State Disaster Medical Advisory Committee*[11]. The chair of that group was contacted about the oxygen issue, and, after discussion with subject matter experts knowledgeable about the delivery of *respiratory therapies*[12], guidance was provided by that evening on the *state DOH website*[13]. The state DOH worked with *emergency management at the State EOC*[14] to airlift additional blood and fluid supplies to the most severely impacted hospitals.

Meanwhile, the jurisdictional EOC has *requested*[15] rotor-wing and ground ambulances from the State EOC to assist with evacuation, and has asked the state to request Federal Disaster Medical Assistance Teams (DMATs). The state has determined that National Disaster Medical System (NDMS) evacuation support for approximately 800 patients who require evacuation from unsafe facilities will be required. This will take days to occur, however, given the broad geographic distribution of severely impacted healthcare facilities, the extent of critical infrastructure disruption, and the time required to mobilize these resources from across the country.

The multiagency *public health and medical emergency support function 8 (ESF-8)*[16] desk at the jurisdictional EOC gets updates on field situations and begins to provide *situational awareness*[17] to the healthcare sector. It is noted during the initial field reports that all 911 services are engaged, affected by the earthquake and *unable to respond or unable to transport*[18] patients.

Hillendale is one of the few functioning trauma centers in the area and, as situational awareness improves, trauma patients are arriving in increasing numbers to Hillendale Hospital. The hospital "clinical care committee" has included *burn and trauma triage information*[19] with its daily recommendations to the incident commander because of this anticipated surge in demand for care. Given that staff surgeons will perform triage based on their clinical judgment, there is no need to activate the plan for a hospital "triage team". This is generally reserved for *tertiary triage of critical care resources*[20], which is not yet an issue.

[21]Clinical Process and Operations: Communication strategies; Clinical Process and Operations: Incident management—jurisdiction

[22]Clinical Process and Operations: Inclusion of palliative care principles

[23]Indicators and Triggers: Critical infrastructure disruption

[24]Indicators and Triggers: Situational awareness

[25]Clinical Process and Operations: Incident management principles

[26]Community and Provider Engagement: Crisis risk communications

[27]Legal Authority and Environment: State and federal declarations

[28]Indicators and Triggers: Illness and injury incidence and severity

[29]Legal Authority and Environment: Medical and legal standards of care

However, the committee *has touched base*[21] with the critical care physicians to assure that they are prepared to implement critical care triage should that be needed. With only a few surgeons available, a few severely burned elderly patients have been *triaged as expectant*[22] and moved to private rooms and made comfortable with analgesia and constant volunteer presence. The hospital continues to have problems notifying staff, who are having problems reaching the facility.

Movement of water, petroleum products, telecommunications, and general transportation repairs will be slow, with many roads and highways impassable in the first few days after the earthquake because of *debris on the roads, damage to bridges, and lack of power*[23] for the traffic signals.

The following morning, *television reports and tweets*[24] are making it clear that thousands of persons have been injured or killed. The state Office of Emergency Management has fully *activated its EOC*[25] and the governor has provided the *media*[26] with an initial briefing. As outlined in the National Response Framework they are attempting to coordinate with the downstate EOCs and mobilize resources to send into the affected area. A *state disaster declaration*[27] has been signed, and a request for federal declaration of disaster has been made and will be approved this morning. Select National Guard assets have been activated. The Health and Human Services Regional Emergency Coordinator has requested the Secretary's Operation Center place the NDMS system on alert, and DMAT activation and patient evacuation planning are in process.

Reports continue to come in to the state EOC that hospitals that are functioning in the affected disaster zone are being inundated with patients seeking care. Hillendale Hospital reports that complete reliance on back-up generator power has limited the number of critical care medical devices that can be supported, while the number of patients requiring critical care interventions continues to rise. Due to the *number and severity of suspected injuries*[28], the state DOH has asked the governor to issue an emergency order authorizing *crisis standards of care*[29] in the affected counties. This order provides additional legal protections to healthcare practitioners and professionals involved in the establishment of and delivery of healthcare services in alternate care sites and shelter environments, which are being set up around the perimeter of the worst affected area.

The "clinical care committee" (which is limited in its ability to contemplate and deliberate on the complete set of issues related to scarcity of resources due to staffing constraints) meets to determine priorities prior to making recommendations to the incident commander at the hospital at 9:00 a.m. Providers are asked to *abandon computer charting*[30] and use simple template charts for minor care. A tent is set up in the parking lot for minor care and is staffed by subspecialty physicians. Intensive care units have overflowed into step-down units. Limited electricity supply continues to affect medical equipment, resulting in some ventilated patients being hand ventilated with use of a bag-valve mask. for prolonged periods of time. Because of the *continued presentation of trauma patients*[31], blood products and surgical supplies are running very low. The requests for assistance to the EOC are repeated, but remain one of many put on hold by the EOC due to more pressing demands.

Later that day, rotor-wing units bring needed supplies and blood from a tertiary care hospital 70 miles north, and take 1 to 2 critical patients back at a time. A large aftershock rattles through the hospital and breaks several more windows. The Planning Chief requests an evacuation list from Operations, which prioritizes existing in-patients for air or ground evacuation and related requirements.

The following day, potable water, generator fuel, and food arrive via National Guard helicopter. The staff is exhausted. That afternoon, members of an internal state disaster response team arrive to begin relieving surgeons and emergency department (ED) physicians. Two days from now, a DMAT team will arrive and set up in an adjacent parking lot, and a larger generator will arrive and be hooked into the hospital electrical supply. Communications is improving. Regional blood supply continues to be tenuous. The "clinical care committee" also has been made aware of very *limited availability of tetanus vaccine*[32], and asks ED staff to vaccinate only for high-risk wounds.

[30]Clinical Process and Operations: Resource-sparing strategies and use of the clinical care committee

[31]Indicators and Triggers: Loss of surge capacity

[32]Clinical Process and Operations: Resource-sparing strategies

[33]Legal Authority and
Environment: Scope of practice

[34]Legal Authority and
Environment: Scope of practice

[35]Clinical Process and
Operations: Recognition of
mental health needs

The State Health Department has also issued *interim guidance*[33] for tetanus vaccine administration in response to this common complaint and is monitoring the daily conference calls and RMCC web-based messaging to identify other issues for the state DOH and the State Disaster Medical Advisory Committee. Fortunately, despite huge demands on the hospital, Hillendale was never forced to appoint a "triage team" or restrict access to critical care resources. Despite seeing 987 patients in the first 3 days, many of the injuries were minor. Although there were a number of severe trauma cases, the general surgery staff helped to *augment*[34] the few trauma surgeons on staff in managing these patients. Twenty-one patients have been airlifted out, the rest remain hospitalized.

The staff are exhausted. Many have lost homes, as have many patients and their family members. Extended family and friends remain unaccounted for or are known to be injured or dead. *Psychological first aid*[35] is provided to victims and staff by trained staff, and social workers try to assist with reunification. The road to recovery will be long and difficult, as the mental health and logistical challenges are just beginning, but Hillendale has played a key part in supporting the needs of the community during this major disaster.

# D

# Workshop Agenda

---

**Guidance for Establishing Standards of Care
for Use in Disaster Situations**

Board on Health Sciences Policy

---

**Public Workshop**

**September 2, 2009**

**Lecture Room
The National Academy of Sciences Building
2100 C Street, NW
Washington, DC**

**Workshop Goals**
- Examine existing standards of care protocols and identify priority elements
- Examine existing guidance for triggers
- Discuss the appropriate balance for guidance versus guidelines. Broad versus granular.

8:00 a.m.        Welcome and Introductions

                        LAWRENCE GOSTIN, *Committee Chair*
                        Associate Dean
                        Research and Academic Programs
                        Director, O'Neill Institute on National and
                            Global Health Law
                        Georgetown University Law Center

                        DAN HANFLING, *Committee Vice-Chair*
                        Special Advisor
                        Emergency Preparedness and Response
                        Inova Health System

8:15             Background and Charge to the Committee

                        RADM ANN KNEBEL
                        Deputy Director for Preparedness and Planning
                        Office of the Assistant Secretary for
                            Preparedness and Response
                        Department of Health and Human Services

8:30             Previous National Accomplishments and Future Needs

                        SALLY PHILLIPS
                        Director
                        Public Health Emergency Preparedness
                        Agency for Healthcare Research and Quality

8:45             Federal Stakeholder Perspectives
                 Panel Objective: Describe relevant federal efforts
                 associated with establishing standards of care. Discuss
                 what national guidance should look like. Discuss what
                 should be included and what should not. Discuss
                 benefits of establishing effective national guidance on
                 standards of care.

                        JON KROHMER
                        Principal Deputy Assistant Secretary and Deputy
                            Chief Medical Officer
                        Office of Health Affairs
                        Department of Homeland Security

CAPT DEBORAH LEVY
Chief, Healthcare Preparedness Activity
Division of Healthcare Quality Promotion
Centers for Disease Control and Prevention

ROGER BERNIER
Associate Director for Science
National Immunization Program
Centers for Disease Control and Prevention

GAMUNU WIJETUNGE
NHTSA/Office of Emergency Medical Services
U.S. Department of Transportation

LTC(P) WAYNE HACHEY
Director Preventive Medicine
Office of the Assistant Secretary of Defense
  (Health Affairs)
Force Health Protection and Readiness

VIRGINIA ASHBY SHARPE
Medical Ethicist
National Center for Ethics in Health Care
Veterans Health Administration

9:30    Discussion with Public Attendees and Committee

10:00   BREAK

10:15   Guidance on Standards of Care in Medical Triage Events
        Panel Objective: Discuss the level of guidance necessary
        during medical triage events. Identify remaining gaps
        limiting the potential effectiveness of existing protocols.

            DAMON ARNOLD, *Panel Chair*
            Director
            Illinois Department of Public Health

            PAUL PATRICK
            Director
            Bureau of EMS and Preparedness
            State of Utah Department of Health

KRISTIN STEVENS
Department of Emergency Management
New York University Langone Medical Center

MEREDITH LI-VOLLMER
Risk Communication Specialist
Seattle and King County Department of Public
 Health

STEVE ROTTMAN
Director
Center for Public Health and Disasters
University of California, Los Angeles

11:15        Discussion with Public Attendees and Committee

11:45        Working Lunch: Continued Discussion with Public
             Attendees and Committee

12:30        Changing Roles and Responsibilities of Healthcare
             Workers under Contingency and Crisis Standards of
             Cares
             Panel Objective: Examine how healthcare worker
             responsibilities change along the standard of care
             continuum. Explore the necessary guidance desired by
             healthcare workers.

             CHERYL PETERSON, *Panel Chair*
             Senior Policy Fellow
             Department of Nursing Practice & Policy
             American Nurses Association

             KRISTINE GEBBIE (note: Via telecon)
             Joan Hansen Grabe Dean
             Hunter-Bellevue School of Nursing

STEVEN LAWRENCE
Associate Director, Emergency Response
Planning
Midwest Regional Center of Excellence for
    Biodefense and Emerging Infectious Diseases
    Research
Assistant Professor of Medicine
Division of Infectious Diseases
Washington University School of Medicine

ROY ALSON
Medical Director, Forsyth County EMS
Medical Director, Disaster Services
North Carolina Office of EMS

MARK GOLDSTEIN
Emergency Services Operations Manager
Emergency Department Memorial Health
System, CO

1:15          Discussion with Public Attendees and Committee

1:45          Guidance on Legal, Ethical, and Practical Issues in
Setting Standards of Care in Declared Emergencies
Panel Discussion: Discuss legal, ethical and practical
issues associated with setting standards of care during
disaster situations. Examine legal distinctions between
standards of care and scope of practice.

JAMES HODGE, *Panel Chair*
Lincoln Professor of Health Law and Ethics
Sandra Day O'Connor College of Law at
Arizona State University

STEPHEN TERET
Professor
Associate Dean; Director
Center for Law and the Public's Health
Johns Hopkins Bloomberg School of Public
    Health

CLIFFORD REES
Research Assistant Professor
Department of Emergency Medicine, Center for
    Disaster Medicine
University of New Mexico School of Medicine

MATTHEW WYNIA
Director of the Institute for Ethics
American Medical Association

MARY ANN BUCKLEY
Senior Attorney
New York State Department of Public Health

2:30          Discussion with Public Attendees and Committee

3:00          Identifying Triggers: Identifying the shift from
              "conventional" to "contingency" and then "crisis" surge
              capacity situations
              Panel Objectives: Discuss the appropriate level of
              guidance and parameters required in the framework for
              guidance from a clinical perspective. Examine how to
              develop guidance so that it matches the available
              resources and evidence-based clinical outcomes, while
              ensuring the greatest number of people saved.

                        JOHN HICK, *Panel Chair*
                        Associate Medical Director for EMS and
                        Medical Director of Emergency Preparedness
                        Hennepin County Medical Center, MN

                        ANTHONY MACINTYRE
                        Associate Professor
                        Department of Emergency Medicine
                        The George Washington University

                        BETSY WEINER (Note: via telecon)
                        Associate Director
                        Nursing Emergency Preparedness Education
                            Coalition
                        Senior Associate Dean, Informatics
                        Vanderbilt University School of Nursing

JAMES GEILING
Associate Professor of Medicine
Dartmouth Medical School

LESLEE STEIN-SPENCER (Note: via telecon)
Manager of Quality Improvement, Chicago Fire
Department
Program Advisor, National Association of State
    EMS Officials

GEORGE TURABELIDZE
Deputy State Epidemiologist
Missouri Department of Health and Senior
Services

BRIAN ERSTAD
Professor and Assistant Department Head
Pharmacy Practice and Science
University of Arizona, College of Pharmacy

4:15    Discussion with Public Attendees and Committee

4:45    Revisiting Overarching Themes: Discussion with Public
        Attendees and Committee

LAWRENCE GOSTIN, *Committee Chair*
Associate Dean
Research and Academic Programs
Director, O'Neill Institute on National and
    Global Health Law
Georgetown University Law Center

DAN HANFLING, *Committee Vice-Chair*
Special Advisor
Emergency Preparedness and Response
Inova Health System

5:30    ADJOURN

# E

# Committee Biographical Information

**Lawrence O. Gostin, J.D., LL.D.** (Hon.) (*Chair*), is an internationally acclaimed scholar in law and public health. He is associate dean (Research and Academic Programs) and the Linda D. and Timothy J. O'Neill Professor of Global Health Law at the Georgetown University Law Center, where he directs the O'Neill Institute for National and Global Health Law. Dean Gostin is also professor of public health at the Johns Hopkins University and director of the Center for Law & the Public's Health at Johns Hopkins and Georgetown Universities—a Collaborating Center of the World Health Organization and the Centers for Disease Control and Prevention (CDC). He is the health law and ethics editor, contributing writer, and columnist for the *Journal of the American Medical Association.* In 2007, the Director General of the World Health Organization appointed Dean Gostin to the International Health Regulations Roster of Experts and the Expert Advisory Panel on Mental Health. Dean Gostin is a member of the Institute of Medicine/National Academy of Sciences, and serves on the Board on Health Sciences Policy and the Committee on Science, Technology, and Law. He has previously chaired committees on health information privacy, genomics, and prisoner research. In the United Kingdom, he was the legal director of the National Association for Mental Health, director of the National Council of Civil Liberties (the U.K. equivalent of the ACLU), and a Fellow at Oxford University. He helped draft the current Mental Health Act (England and Wales) and brought several landmark cases before the European Commission and Court of Human Rights. Dean Gostin has led major U.S. law reform initiatives, including the drafting of the Model Emergency Health Powers Act to combat bioterrorism and the "Turning Point" Model State Public Health Act. He is also leading a drafting team on developing a Model Public Health Law for the World Health Organization.

**Dan Hanfling, M.D.** (*Vice Chair*), is special advisor to the Inova Health System in Falls Church, VA, on matters related to emergency preparedness and disaster response. He is a board-certified emergency physician practicing at Inova Fairfax Hospital, Northern Virginia's Level 1 trauma center. He serves as an operational medical director for PHI Air Medical Group—Virginia, the largest private rotor-wing air medevac service in Virginia, and has responsibilities as a medical team manager for Virginia Task Force One, an international urban search and rescue team sanctioned by FEMA and USAID. He has been involved in the response to international and domestic disasters, including the Izmit, Turkey, earthquake in 1999; the Pentagon terrorism incident on September 11, 2001; Hurricanes Rita and Katrina in 2005; and Hurricanes Gustav and Ike in 2008. Dr. Hanfling was intricately involved in the management of the response to the anthrax bioterrorism mailings in the fall of 2001, when two cases of inhalational anthrax were successfully diagnosed at Inova Fairfax Hospital. Dr. Hanfling received an A.B. in Political Science from Duke University and was awarded his M.D. from Brown University. He completed an internship in Internal Medicine at the Miriam Hospital in Providence, RI, and an Emergency Medicine Residency at George Washington and Georgetown University Hospitals. He is a clinical professor of Emergency Medicine at George Washington University and an invited member of the George Mason University School of Public Policy Advisory Board.

**Damon T. Arnold, M.D., M.P.H.,** was named the 16th director of the Illinois Department of Public Health on October 1, 2007. Prior to his current position, Dr. Arnold was the medical director for bioterrorism and preparedness for the Chicago Department of Public Health. During his professional career, he was also medical director for St. Francis Hospital, Blue Island, IL; LTV Steel Company in Indiana; and Mercy Hospital and Medical Center, Chicago. He has served in the Army National Guard for 25 years, holds the rank of Colonel and currently is the Guard's commander of the Joint Task Force Medical Command in Springfield and the Illinois State Surgeon. Over the years, he has had a distinguished military career and received many military awards, including Army Commendation, National Defense Service and Humanitarian Service medals. He has served missions to Iraq, Kuwait,

Central America, South America, Africa, and Europe, as well as participated in relief efforts for Hurricanes Katrina and Rita. He was the American Red Cross Military Hero of the Year for 2007. Dr. Arnold received his M.D. and M.P.H. degrees from the University of Illinois, and has completed several law courses at DePaul University College of Law. Dr. Arnold chairs the Association of State and Territorial Health Officials (ASTHO) Preparedness Policy Committee, sits on the Board of Directors for the American Red Cross of Greater Chicago, and serves as ASTHO Liaison Representative for the Board of Scientific Counselors, Coordinating Office for Terrorism Preparedness and Emergency Response. Dr. Arnold also holds associate professorships at the University of Illinois School of Public Health, the University of Illinois Medical School, and the Southern Illinois Medical School.

**Stephen V. Cantrill, M.D., FACEP,** is an emergency physician from Denver, CO, who recently retired from serving as the associate director of Emergency Medicine at Denver Health Medical Center for 18 years. He was also the director of the Colorado BNICE WMD Training Program at Denver Health for more than 5 years. Dr. Cantrill has lectured nationally and internationally on many topics, including weapons of mass destruction, disasters, and disaster management, and has been involved in disaster management education for more than two decades. He served as the regional medical coordinator for Denver's participation in Operation TopOff 2000. He has also been involved in weapons of mass destruction training for Colorado and has participated in the planning for multiple mass-gathering events, including the Denver visit by the Pope and the Denver Summit of Eight world economic conference. He has testified at U.S. Senate Committee hearings on bioterrorism preparedness. He recently served as the principal investigator on an Agency for Healthcare Research and Quality (AHRQ) regional surge capacity grant and the AHRQ HAvBED national bed availability project. He also served as principal investigator on the AHRQ disaster alternate care facility task order. Dr. Cantrill has more than 90 publications to his credit and has been the recipient of multiple teaching and clinical excellence awards.

**Brooke Courtney, J.D., M.P.H.,** is an associate at the Center for Biosecurity of UPMC. Ms. Courtney's research focuses on public health and hospital preparedness, legal preparedness, and mass dispensing of medical countermeasures. She is an associate editor of the peer-reviewed journal, *Biosecurity and Bioterrorism: Biodefense Strategy, Practice, and Science*, and editor of the journal's Legal Perspectives column. Prior to joining the Center, Ms. Courtney served as director of the Office of Public Health Preparedness and Response for the Baltimore City Health Department, where she provided oversight of the city's responses to public health emergencies. Previously, she worked on surge capacity and pandemic influenza planning with the University of Maryland Center for Health and Homeland Security. She has also worked as a Law Fellow for the U.S. Senate Committee on Health, Education, Labor, and Pensions and for the Public Health Division of the U.S. Department of Health and Human Services' Office of the General Counsel, as well as a Law Clerk in the Health Fraud Division of the U.S. Attorney's Office for the District of Maryland. In addition, Ms. Courtney has worked on international relations and disaster response at the American Red Cross national headquarters; on outcomes research at Pfizer Inc.; on issues related to healthcare coverage at the Maryland Health Care Commission; and on tobacco control, obesity, and health disparities issues. Ms. Courtney received her J.D. and certificate in health law from the University of Maryland School of Law and is admitted to practice in Maryland. She received her M.P.H. from Yale University, and is a Phi Beta Kappa graduate of the University of Colorado at Boulder.

**Asha Devereaux, M.D., M.P.H.,** is a pulmonary/critical care physician in private practice in Coronado, CA. Dr. Devereaux has 11 years of training and service with the U.S. Navy and formerly served as the intensive care unit director on the isolation unit of the USNS Mercy Hospital ship. She currently serves as a Steering Committee Member for the American College of Chest Physicians Disaster Response Network. Dr. Devereaux has spearheaded a national conference on disaster preparedness, has published on the topic, and presently serves on the California State Board of the American Lung Association. Dr. Devereaux is also president of the California Thoracic Society and the lead physician advisor of the San Diego Medical Reserve Corps. Dr. Devereaux received her undergraduate education at the University of California–San Diego, followed by her M.D./M.P.H. from Tulane University.

**Edward J. Gabriel, M.P.A., AEMT-P,** is director, Global Crisis Management, for The Walt Disney Company, and is responsible for the development and implementation of global policy, planning, training, and exercises to manage crises for The Walt Disney Company. He is also responsible for East and West Coast Medical and Emergency Medical Operations and the Walt Disney Studio's Fire Department. He supports and collaborates with global business units in development and testing of resumption planning, and develops policies and strategies to manage crises. Mr. Gabriel has been an emergency medical technician (EMT) since 1973 and was a 27-year paramedic veteran of the New York City Fire Department's Emergency Medical Service. He rose through the ranks from EMT to paramedic through lieutenant and retired at the level of assistant chief/division commander. As deputy commissioner for planning and preparedness at the New York City Office of Emergency Management, he served as commissioner for all preparedness and planning-related projects and initiatives. During his role with New York City, he was a member of the Federal Bureau of Investigation/New York City Joint Terrorism Task Force (JTTF), and still sits on the International Advisory Board of the *Journal of Emergency Care, Rescue and Transportation*. He has worked with The Joint Commission, sitting on the Emergency Preparedness Roundtable as well as the Community Linkages in Bioterrorism Preparedness Expert Panel. He served as a member of the U.S. Department of Health and Human Services (HHS) Federal Contingency Medical Facility Working Group and the AHRQ Expert Panel on Mass Casualty Medical Care. Most recently he has worked with the AHRQ expert panel as principal author of the prehospital chapter of the *Providing Mass Medical Care with Scarce Resources: Community Planning Guide* and with the U.S. Department of Defense, General George C. Marshall School of International Studies Program on Terrorism and Security Studies, located in Garmisch-Partenkirchen, Germany, presenting on methodologies for planning and preparedness for international leaders. He is credentialed through the International Association of Emergency Managers as a Certified Emergency Manager and the Disaster Recovery Institute International as a Certified Business Continuity Professional. Mr. Gabriel holds a B.A. from the College of New Rochelle and an M.P.A. from Rutgers University. Mr. Gabriel continues to lecture nationally and internationally on crisis management, business continuity, emergency management, planning and preparedness, WMD, terrorism, and emergency medical topics.

**John L. Hick, M.D.,** is a faculty emergency physician at Hennepin County Medical Center (HCMC) and an associate professor of

Emergency Medicine at the University of Minnesota. He serves as the associate medical director for Hennepin County Emergency Medical Services and Medical Director for Emergency Preparedness at HCMC. He is medical advisor to the Minneapolis/St. Paul Metropolitan Medical Response System. He also serves the Minnesota Department of Health as the medical director for both the Office of Emergency Preparedness and Hospital Bioterrorism Preparedness. He is the founder and past chair of the Minneapolis/St. Paul Metropolitan Hospital Compact, a 29-hospital mutual aid and planning group active since 2002. He is involved at many levels of planning for surge capacity and adjusted standards of care and traveled to Greece to assist in healthcare system preparations for the 2004 Summer Olympics as part of a 15-member CDC/HHS team. He is a national speaker on hospital preparedness issues and has published numerous papers dealing with hospital preparedness for contaminated casualties, personal protective equipment, and surge capacity.

**James G. Hodge, Jr., J.D., LL.M.,** is the Lincoln Professor of Health Law and Ethics at the Sandra Day O'Connor College of Law and Fellow, Center for the Study of Law, Science, and Technology, at Arizona State University (ASU). He is also a senior scholar at the Centers for Law and the Public's Health: A Collaborative at Johns Hopkins and Georgetown Universities and current president of the Public Health Law Association. Prior to joining ASU in August 2009, he was a professor at the Johns Hopkins Bloomberg School of Public Health; adjunct professor of law at Georgetown University Law Center; executive director of the Centers for Law and the Public's Health; and a core faculty member of the Johns Hopkins Berman Institute of Bioethics. Through his scholarly and applied work, Professor Hodge delves into multiple areas of public health law, global health law, ethics, and human rights. The recipient of the 2006 Henrik L. Blum Award for Excellence in Health Policy from the American Public Health Association, he has drafted (with others) several public health law reform initiatives, including the Model State Public Health Information Privacy Act, the Model State Emergency Health Powers Act, the Turning Point Model State Public Health Act, and the Uniform Emergency Volunteer Health Practitioners Act. His diverse, funded projects include work on (1) the legal framework underlying the use of volunteer health professionals during emergencies; (2) the compilation, study, and analysis of state genetics laws and policies as part of a multiyear National Institutes of Health-funded project; (3) historical and legal bases underlying school vaccination programs; (4) international tobacco policy for the World Health Organization's Tobacco Free Initiative; (5) legal and ethical distinctions between public health practice and research; (6) legal underpinnings of partner notification and expedited partner therapies; and (7) public health law case studies in multiple states. He is a national expert on public health information privacy law and ethics, having consulted with HHS, CDC, FDA, CMS, OHRP, APHA, CSTE, APHL, and others on privacy issues.

**Donna E. Levin, J.D.,** is the general counsel for the Massachusetts Department of Public Health. Prior to her appointment in 1988, Ms. Levin served as a deputy general counsel and concentrated in several different areas of health law, including determination of need, long-term care and hospital regulation, and environmental health. In her current role, she manages the Office of General Counsel and advises the Commissioner of Public Health and senior staff on all legal aspects concerning the implementation of Department responsibilities pursuant to statutory and regulatory authority; major policy initiatives of the Department; and legislation affecting the Department's interests. Most recently, Ms. Levin has focused on the expansion of newborn screening services in Massachusetts; the review and analysis of the Massachusetts Law on Genetics and Privacy; implementation of the Health Insurance Consumer Protections Law; issues of public health authority and emergency response; and legal oversight of eight professional health boards. Ms. Levin is a member of the Health Law Section Steering Committee of the Boston Bar Association. She holds a B.A. from the State University of New York at Stony Brook and a J.D. from Northeastern University School of Law.

**Marianne Matzo, Ph.D., GNP-BC, FPCN, FAAN,** is professor and Endowed Ziegler Chair in Palliative Care Nursing in the College of Nursing and adjunct professor, Department of Geriatric Medicine, at the University of Oklahoma Health Sciences Center. Dr. Matzo is director of the Sooner Palliative Care Institute, through which research is conducted to ensure the delivery of high-quality care and to educate health professionals. She has received research funding from the American Cancer Society and the Oncology Nursing Society to conduct research related to sexual health issues in the palliative care population. She was a 2008 Recipient of the Project on Death in America Nursing Leadership Award in Palliative Care sponsored by the Hospice and Palliative Nurses

Foundation. Dr. Matzo is a nationally and internationally recognized palliative care educator who has developed and taught educational programs in Japan, Russia, and Serbia. In addition, Dr. Matzo is a three-time winner of the *American Journal of Nursing* Book of the Year award. Dr. Matzo has published in numerous peer-reviewed publications and is involved in ongoing work in disaster planning for situations in which there are scarce resources.

**Cheryl A. Peterson, M.S.N., R.N.,** is the director of Nursing Practice and Policy at the American Nurses Association (ANA). Prior to that, she was a senior policy fellow for the ANA, responsible for researching and developing association policy related to preparing for and responding to a disaster, whether manmade or natural. Since 1998, Ms. Peterson has been actively involved in disaster planning at the federal level. In addition, she coordinated the ANA's response to the tsunami in Southeast Asia and to hurricanes during the 2005 U.S. hurricane season. Ms. Peterson spent 13 years in the Reserve Army Nurse Corps and in 1990 was deployed during Desert Storm. She also spent 7 years as an active volunteer in the Kensington, MD, Volunteer Fire Department. Ms. Peterson received her B.S.N. from the University of Cincinnati and her M.S.N. from Georgetown University.

**Tia Powell, M.D.,** is director of the Montefiore-Einstein Center for Bioethics and a faculty member at Albert Einstein College of Medicine and the Montefiore Medical Center in New York. She served from 2004 to 2008 as executive director of the New York State Task Force on Life and the Law and from 1992 to 1998 as director of Clinical Ethics at Columbia-Presbyterian Hospital in New York City. She is a graduate of Harvard-Radcliffe College and Yale Medical School. She did her psychiatric internship, residency, and a fellowship in Consultation-Liaison Psychiatry all at Columbia University, College of P&S, and the New York State Psychiatric Institute. She is a Fellow of the American Psychiatric Association and of the New York Academy of Medicine and a member of the American Society of Bioethics and Humanities. In 2007, she co-chaired the New York State Department of Health's workgroup to develop guidelines for allocating ventilators during a flu pandemic.

**Merritt Schreiber, Ph.D.,** is senior manager for Psychological Programs and associate research psychologist in the Center for Public Health and

Disasters, School of Public Health at the University of California–Los Angeles Center for the Health Sciences. Dr. Schreiber's current academic work is focused on the development of public health approaches to the mental health consequences of catastrophic events. He has developed the first known disaster mental-health rapid-triage system, "PsySTART," for the American Red Cross and Los Angeles County Level 1 trauma centers. Dr. Schreiber has also developed disaster mental health core competencies for the state of California, a model state plan for mental health response to pandemic influenza, and is currently working on a catastrophic event mental health concept of operations for Los Angeles County. Dr. Schreiber was appointed to the Secretary's Emergency Public Information and Communications Advisory Board, where he worked on policy recommendations on the risk communications for our nation, and particularly the needs of children and families, for the Secretary of HHS. Dr. Schreiber is also the University of California Office of the President representative to the State of California Department of Public Health Emergency Preparedness Office Joint Advisory Committee, and was a member of the California public health emergency preparedness planning project in this role. Dr. Schreiber was a first responder to Hurricane Katrina during two tours as a reserved commissioned officer with the U.S. Public Health Service and as mental health team lead with California Disaster Medical Assistance Team CA-1, National Disaster Medical System (NDMS), where he was also a member of the NDMS Senior Medical Working Group. He received a presidential citation from the American Psychological Association for his work with victims' families after 9/11 and received the Outstanding Humanitarian Contribution Award from the California Psychological Association in 2004.

**Umair A. Shah, M.D., M.P.H.,** has served as deputy director of Harris County Public Health & Environmental Services (HCPHES) and director of the HCPHES Disease Control & Clinical Prevention Division since 2004. HCPHES is the county health department for the Houston area, offering an array of population-based public health services. Harris County is the third most populous county in the United States (3.98 million), spanning more than 1,700 square miles and encompassing a vastly diverse community. Originally from Cincinnati, OH, Dr. Shah received his undergraduate philosophy degree with an interest in medical ethics from Vanderbilt University. He then went on to obtain his MD from The University of Toledo Health Science Center, where he was also

selected for an International Health & Public Policy Internship at the World Health Organization headquarters in Geneva, Switzerland. Dr. Shah then completed his residency in Internal Medicine, fellowship in Primary Care/General Medicine, and his M.P.H., all at The University of Texas Health Science Center at Houston. Upon completion of training, he served several years as an emergency department attending physician at Houston's Michael E. DeBakey VA Medical Center before becoming the chief medical officer at the Galveston County Health District. Dr. Shah's interests include international and refugee health, emergency/disaster response, and health equity-related work. His large-scale disaster experiences include responses related to Tropical Storm Allison; Hurricanes Katrina, Rita, and Ike; and the Kashmir earthquake. He currently serves on the National Association of County and City Health Officials (NACCHO) Health Equity and Social Justice Team, the NACCHO International Public Health Workgroup, and the Board of Directors for the South Asian Public Health Association. He was recently selected to serve on the Second National Consensus Panel on Emergency Preparedness and Cultural Diversity sponsored by the HHS Office of Minority Health. Dr. Shah is a writer who has co-authored many peer-reviewed journal articles in public health and remains engaged in teaching as an adjunct faculty member of the University of Texas School of Public Health. He is board certified in internal medicine, remains active in clinical patient care, and serves as one of the local health authorities for Harris County.